Male Depression, Alcoholism and Violence

D0147363

Male Depression, Alcoholism and Violence

Ihsan M Salloum MD, MPH
Associate Professor of Psychiatry
Medical Director, Center for Psychiatric and Chemical Dependency Services (CPCDS)

Dennis C Daley PhD
Associate Professor of Psychiatry
Chief, Drug and Alcohol Services

Michael E Thase MD
Professor of Psychiatry
Chief, Division of Adult Academic Psychiatry

University of Pittsburgh Medical Center Health System
Western Psychiatric Institute and Clinic
Pittsburgh
PA 15213
USA

MARTIN DUNITZ

The views expressed in this publication are
those of the authors and do not necessarily
reflect those of Martin Dunitz Ltd

© Martin Dunitz Ltd 2000

First published in the United Kingdom in 2000 by
Martin Dunitz Ltd
The Livery House
7–9 Pratt Street
London NW1 0AE

Tel:	+44 (0)207 482 2202
Fax:	+44 (0)207 267 0159
E-mail:	info@mdunitz.globalnet.co.uk
Website:	http://www.dunitz.co.uk

A CIP catalogue record for this book is
available from the British Library

ISBN 1–85317–894–2

Distributed in the USA, Canada and Brazil by:

Blackwell Science Inc.
Commerce Place, 350 Main Street
Malden MA 02148, USA
Tel: 1 800 215 1000

Printed and bound in Italy

Contents

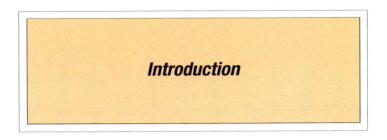

Introduction

Public health significance

Depression and alcoholism are among the most frequent disorders found in community surveys and clinical studies.[1,2] These disorders, alone and in combination, are associated with a multiplicity of adverse medical, psychological, family, economic and spiritual consequences.[3,4] Patients with these dual disorders are also overrepresented in mental health or substance abuse treatment systems, as individuals suffering from more than one condition are more likely to seek help.[5]

Violence is also a significant problem among some individuals with psychiatric disorders[6–8] and alcoholism or other substance use disorders.[9,10] Violent behaviours such as homicide, assaults and domestic violence cause considerable suffering for families and society. Patients with violence problems may enter treatment primarily for help with alcoholism or other substance abuse, a mood disorder, or other type of psychiatric disorder. These patients often do not recognize their violence as a problem that needs changing and enter treatment as a result of external pressures from the family, legal system or caregivers.

The purpose of this book is to help physicians and health care providers understand alcoholism, depression and violence among men. We will discuss prevalence of these problems, the assessment process, treatment engagement, pharmacotherapy, psychosocial treatments and maintenance or relapse prevention strategies.

Prevalence of depression and alcoholism in men

Studies show a higher frequency of alcoholism among males and a higher frequency of depression among females.[1-4,11,12] One large epidemiological study found that 24% of men with alcohol dependence had major depression during their lifetime, a rate three times that of the general population. Depression among women with alcohol dependence was reported at 48.5%, a rate four times that of the general population.[11] In psychiatric settings, up to 34% of depressed patients have alcoholism while 24–59% of patients in alcoholism treatment have depression.[13-20]

Impact of dual disorders

Many individual, family and societal problems are associated with depression, alcoholism and/or violence.[21-23] Alcoholism confounds the diagnostic picture of depression, interferes with treatment compliance, completion and response to medications or therapy, increases the risk of suicidal or violent behaviours, increases the rate of costly medical and psychiatric health service utilization, and is a factor in rehospitalization.[24-29] These problems cause considerable suffering for the family system and individual members, and contribute to marital and family break-up.[23,30]

Symptom presentation and associated comorbidities

- Increased suicidal and aggressive behaviour
- Polysymptomatic presentation
- High prevalence of other drugs of abuse
- High prevalence of personality disorders
- High prevalence of medical disorders
- High prevalence of HIV risk behaviour
- Increased violent and criminal behaviour
- Poor psychosocial and family functioning

Health service use

- Increased hospital admission rates
- Longer hospital stays
- Increased use of other expensive medical services (e.g. emergency room)

Treatment response

- Poor treatment adherence
- Poor response to treatment
- Increased risk of relapse to alcohol or other drugs
- Increased rate of relapse to depression
- Increased rate of psychiatric rehospitalization

Table 1
Symptoms and problems related to comorbid alcoholism, depression and violence

Violence among depressed males with alcohol dependence

Violence and alcoholism

The association between violent behaviour, alcoholism and male gender is well documented.[31] Violence is also reported to be high among community depressed patients.[32]

Several factors contribute to the association between alcohol abuse and violent behaviour, especially among males.

Direct effects of alcohol on the central nervous system lead to impairment in the capacity of self-regulation by disrupting the Executive Cognitive Functioning (ECF) of the prefrontal cortex.[33] Impairment in ECF is related to aggression and delinquent behaviour.[34] High levels of testosterone[35,36] appear to interact with alcohol intoxication to increase aggression.[37]

Studies have found a dose–response relationship between violence-related injuries and alcohol consumption. Quantity, rather than frequency, of alcohol drinking predicts violent behaviour.[38] There is some evidence that violent and aggressive behaviours are related to the raising of blood alcohol levels, rather than to the decreasing blood alcohol levels after a bout of drinking alcohol.[39]

Individual vulnerabilities include traits such as sensation seeking,[40] impaired impulse control[41] and psychopathology such as conduct disorder or antisocial personality disorder.[42] For example, antisocial personality disorder may overlap with Cloningers' type II alcoholism, a type of alcoholism found among males who usually have early onset of alcohol problems and involvement in antisocial behaviours.[43]

Social and cultural factors mediating alcohol-induced violence range from an environment that promotes or contributes to deviant behaviour or a violent lifestyle,[40] to social expectancy of aggression as an effect of alcohol intoxication.[44]

Alcohol-related factors

Direct effect of alcohol on the central nervous system:

- Disinhibition hypothesis: alcohol disrupts self-regulation abilities by weakening those mechanisms that usually restrain impulsive and aggressive behaviour, e.g. the Executive Cognitive Functioning (ECF)
- Alcohol impairs cognitive processing, e.g. leading patients to misjudge social cues, thereby overreacting to a perceived threat
- Alcohol causes narrowing of attention, which may lead to an inaccurate assessment of the future risk of acting on an immediate violent impulse

Individual vulnerabilities:

- Temperamental traits, such as sensation-seeking personalities
- Impaired impulse control
- Associated psychopathology such as conduct disorder, antisocial personality disorders and intermittent explosive disorder
- Impairment in ECF predating the onset of alcohol misuse
- Serotonergic system dysfunction
- High levels of testosterone

Social and cultural factors mediating alcohol-induced violence

- Expectancy of violence with alcohol intoxication
- Deviant behaviour and violent lifestyle

Depression-related factors

Symptoms of agitation and anxiety
The presence of 'anger attacks'

Table 2
Risk factors for violent behaviour in depressed males with alcohol dependence

Violence and depression

In depressed patients, anger and aggression have been linked to symptoms of agitation and anxiety.[45] More recently, 'anger attacks' have been found to be associated with major depressive disorders.[46] Dysregulated anger is a sudden and intense 'attack' of anger highly disproportionate to the stimulus provocation. Anger attacks are more frequent among depressed patients compared to normal controls[47] and among depressed males compared to depressed females.[48]

Suicidality

Patients with comorbid depression and alcoholism are among the highest risk psychiatric patients for suicidal behaviour.[49] Major depression and alcohol dependence are the major leading causes of completed suicide with lifetime rates of 15% for major depression, and a risk of suicide for the alcohol dependent estimated at 60–120 times higher than that of the general population.[50] The risk of suicide increases when the two disorders co-exist. Studies of clinical populations find that the intensity of suicidal behaviour is among the most salient distinguishing characteristics of comorbid depression and alcoholism compared to either depression or alcohol dependence alone.[4,26] Suicidal behaviour is also a major leading cause of psychiatric hospitalization for these patients. Alcohol use is very common prior to attempting or completing suicide.[29] The quantity of alcohol consumed correlates with suicide attempts among depressed patients with alcohol dependence[51] and non-depressed such patients.[52] Heavy alcohol use increased the risk of death by suicide by six times in a community sample.[53] There are few premeditated suicide attempts among depressed patients with alcohol dependence as they usually use the most easily available method.[51]

Serotonergic system dysfunction and alcoholism, depression, violence and suicide

Serotonergic system dysfunction is thought to underlie depression, alcoholism, alcohol-induced aggression, suicide, impulsivity, aggression and violence.[54] Serotonergic system dysfunction distinguishes subgroups of depressed patients who report 'anger attacks'.[55] Serotonin is thought to function as a behavioural inhibitor. A decrease in serotonin activity is associated with increased aggressiveness and impulsivity[35,56] and with early-onset alcoholism among men.[57] Animal studies[58] indicate that central serotonin dysfunction is associated with lower initial sensitivity to alcohol intoxication with greater aggression. Parental neglect leads to early onset aggression and excessive alcohol consumption in offspring, and is correlated with decreased serotonin activity.[57] Other neurotransmitters such as dopamine and norepinephrine may mediate the alcohol–violence link as well.[59]

Introduction

The goals of the initial assessment are to formulate diagnoses, develop an initial treatment plan, and determine the type and intensity of treatment services needed, including the need for detoxification or psychiatric hospitalization. Another important goal is to assess the patient's level of motivation and receptiveness to treatment.

Patients with depression, alcoholism and/or violence problems often have multiple difficulties including other psychiatric and personality disorders, high levels of social stressors, physical disorders and impaired functioning.[4] The multiaxial formulations of both the DSM-IV and the ICD-10 diagnostic systems provide a useful format to record clinical diagnoses and functional difficulties presented by these patients.[60,61]

Axis I: Clinical disorders

- Substance use, cognitive, psychotic, mood, anxiety, somatoform, factitous, dissociative, sexual and gender identity, eating, sleep impulse control and adjustment disorders, etc.

Axis II: Personality disorders

- Prominent maladaptive personality features or defence mechanisms
- Mental retardation

Axis III: General medical conditions

Axis IV: Psychosocial and environmental problems

- Primary support groups
- Social environment
- Educational
- Occupational
- Housing
- Economic
- Access to health care
- Legal
- Other problems

Axis V: Global assessment of functioning

Table 3
DSM-IV multiaxial formulation

Assessment of alcohol use disorders

Alcohol dependence refers to a 'cluster of cognitive, behavioral, and physiological symptoms indicating that the individual continues to use alcohol despite significant alcohol-related problems'.[62] Core elements include the loss of control over drinking behaviour as manifested by a narrowing of the drinking repertoire, compulsion to drink and alcohol-seeking behaviour, the presence of physiological dependence and the rapid reinstatement of the dependence syndrome after a period of abstinence.[63] The DSM-IV diagnostic system requires that three out of seven criteria be present at any time within the same 12-month period to meet the diagnosis of alcohol dependence. This is further specified with or without physiological dependence based on the evidence of tolerance and withdrawal.[62] Alcohol abuse refers to a 'maladaptive pattern of alcohol use, occurring within a 12-month period, and leading to recurrent and significant adverse consequences, and which have never met the criteria for alcohol dependence'.

Alcohol use disorders	Alcohol-induced disorders
Alcohol abuse Alcohol dependence ***Specifiers*** • With physiological dependence • Without physiological dependence • Early partial remission • Early full remission • Sustained partial remission • Sustained full remission • On agonist therapy • In a controlled environment	• Intoxication • Withdrawal • Intoxication delirium • Withdrawal delirium • Persisting dementia • Persisting amnesic disorder • Psychotic disorder, with delusion • Psychotic disorder, with hallucination • Mood disorder • Anxiety disorder • Sexual dysfunction • Sleep disorder

Table 4
DSM-IV diagnoses for alcohol-related disorders

Alcohol dependence	Alcohol abuse
• Tolerance • Withdrawal • Alcohol taken in larger amount or over a longer period than was intended • Persistent desire or unsuccessful efforts to cut down or control use • A great deal of time is spent on activities necessary to obtain alcohol • Important social, occupational or recreational activities are given up or reduced because of alcohol use • Alcohol use is continued despite knowledge of having a persistent or recurrent physical or psychological problem caused or exacerbated by alcohol	• Recurrent alcohol use resulting in a failure to fulfil major role obligations at work, school or home • Recurrent use of alcohol in situations in which it is physically hazardous • Recurrent alcohol-related legal problems • Continued alcohol use despite having persistent or recurrent social or interpersonal problems caused or exacerbated by the effects of alcohol

Table 5
DSM-IV alcohol use disorders

Initial diagnostic assessment

Following are key elements of a comprehensive initial diagnostic assessment for patients with an alcohol use disorder, depressive disorder and/or violence.

- Patient interview
- Informant interview (significant others, referring agencies, other health providers)
- Signs and symptoms of alcoholism and major depression
- Mental status examination
- Medical information review
- Physical examination
- Laboratory tests
- Blood alcohol concentration (BAC)/breath alcohol levels (BAL), urine drug screen, other laboratory tests
- History of current and past stress, medical, occupational, social, legal problems and family history
- The use of screening instruments, rating scales and structured clinical interviews

Table 6
Key elements of an initial diagnostic assessment

Patient interview

While patients usually feel comfortable discussing depressive symptoms, eliciting a history of alcohol or drug abuse, or a history of violence may generate defensiveness, particularly among patients who deny or minimize their problem. A non-judgemental and matter-of-fact approach can help reduce defensiveness and facilitate compliance with treatment recommendations.[64]

An assessment of alcohol use history includes a review of the quantity and frequency of all substances currently and previously used, and the presence of tolerance and withdrawal complications, or the presence of adverse psychological, medical, interpersonal, social, vocational, financial, spiritual or legal consequences. Assessment should also include the presence of obsessions and compulsions to use, attempts to cut down or stop, and experiences with relapse.[65]

Other interviews

Informant or collateral interviews with family members, significant others, or health care professionals can often provide additional information about the patient. Family and significant others can also play a significant role in the recovery process by influencing the patient to seek and comply with treatment, and providing support.[66]

Physical examination

A physical examination and a comprehensive medical history are important to assess signs of alcohol intoxication or withdrawal, medical consequences of alcohol or drug use, and to rule out medical problems that can complicate the alcohol withdrawal syndrome. Alcohol withdrawal complications, such as seizures or delirium tremens, are more likely to occur in those with compromised physical health.

Laboratory tests

Initial drug screening can help rule out the likelihood of alcohol or drug overdose. Breath alcohol levels (BAL) or blood alcohol concentration (BAC) provide objective measurements of the intoxication state and the levels of tolerance. For example, a BAL of 200–300 mg/ml in a patient who displays only minor signs of intoxication indicates high levels of tolerance and likelihood of severe withdrawal syndrome.[67] These tests are also useful during treatment to monitor alcohol and other substance use. An initial test battery may include urine analysis, complete blood count with differential, blood chemistry, serology and liver enzymes. Hepatitis screening and HIV testing should also be performed in high-risk groups, such as those with other drug use, especially intravenous drug users of heroin, and cocaine and crack cocaine users.

Assessment instruments

These provide a validated approach to the identification and diagnosis of alcohol-related disorders. Assessment instruments can also be used in treatment planning and in assessing the treatment process and outcome. The publication *Assessing Alcohol Problems: A Guide for Clinicians and Researchers*[68] is an excellent resource on the subject. Commonly used assessment instruments are given below.

Screening instruments (10 items or fewer):
- Alcohol Use Disorder Identification Test (AUDIT)
- CAGE questionnaire
- The Brief Michigan Alcoholism Screening Test (MAST)

Diagnostic rating scales:
- Alcohol Dependence Scale (ADS)
- Severity of Alcohol Dependence Questionnaire (SADQ)
- Clinical Institute Withdrawal Assessment Scale for Alcohol-revised (CIWA-r)

Structured diagnostic interviews:
- Structured Clinical Interview for DSM-IV (SCID)
- Psychiatric Research Interview for Substance and Mental Disorders (PRISM)

Assessment of drinking behaviour:
- Alcohol Timeline Followback (TLFB)
- Drinking Self-Monitoring Log (DSML)[69]
- Lifetime Drinking History (LDH)[70]

Treatment planning, treatment process and outcome evaluation:
- Addiction Severity Index (ASI)
- Alcohol Use Inventory[71]
- Inventory of Drinking Situations (IDS)[72]
- Alcohol-Specific Role Play Test (ASRPT)
- Treatment Services Review (TSR)[73]
- Drinker Inventory of Consequences (DrInC)
- Follow-up Drinker Profile (FDP)[74]

Table 7
Assessment instruments

Screening instruments

There are a number of simple, time-efficient, reliable and widely used pen and paper screening instruments to assess alcohol problems such as the CAGE questionnaire,[75] the Brief Michigan Alcoholism Screening Test (MAST)[76] and the Alcohol Use Disorder Identification Test (AUDIT).[77] The CAGE is a very brief, 4-item, widely used screening instrument, while AUDIT is a 10-item questionnaire that provides information on the amount and frequency, the alcohol dependence syndrome, and on problems caused by alcohol.

Rating scales and structured diagnostic interviews

The Alcohol Dependence Scale (ADS)[78] and the Severity of Alcohol Dependence Questionnaire (SADQ)[79] provide a measure of the severity of the dependence syndrome. The Structured Clinical Interview for DSM-IV (SCID)[80] and the Psychiatric Research Interview for Substance and Mental Disorders (PRISM)[81] provide reliable DSM-IV psychiatric diagnoses. These instruments, however, are very time consuming, although primary care versions of the SCID are now available.[82]

Other instruments, such as the Alcohol Timeline Followback (TLFB),[83] the Addiction Severity Index (ASI),[84] Alcohol-Specific Role Play Test (ASRPT)[85] and Drinker Inventory of Consequences (DrInC)[86] assess drinking behaviour, treatment planning, treatment process, and treatment outcome. For example, the ASI provides indices of severity in seven health-related domains including alcohol, other drugs, psychiatric, medical, family, social and legal areas. The ASI also provides a measure of change over time in terms of severity and frequency of alcohol and drug use.

Assessment of alcohol withdrawal

The Clinical Institute Withdrawal Assessment Scale for Alcohol-Revised version (CIWA-r) provides a comprehensive assessment of the withdrawal syndrome and it requires approximately 5–7 minutes to administer.[87] Versions of this instrument have been found to be useful in dual diagnosis patients as well.[88]

Assessment of depression

Depression involves somatic, mood and behavioural symptoms. Depression among males may also involve anger, irritability, hostility and violent behaviour, and there is evidence that alcohol and other drug abuse may influence the probability of such dyscontrol. Obviously, cultural standards influence the expression of depression. Some investigators have pointed out that males may differ from females in their style of response to the presence of depression. While females are more likely to show a 'ruminative' style, with increased focus on their emotional states, men are more likely to have a 'distracting' response.[89] Males are more likely to focus on distracting tasks not related to depression; the distracting style is thought to be more effective than the ruminative style in coping with depression. However, males are also more likely to develop maladaptive distracting activities such as alcohol use. Alcohol misuse may then develop into alcohol-related problems.[90,91] Furthermore, males and females may differ in their expression of emotional distress such as that induced by depression. For example, studies of chronic depression among adolescents reported that males were more aggressive and antagonistic than females.[92] They may also differ in gender-specific socializing experiences such as the quality of their relationships.

On the other hand, more recent, large, multicentre studies failed to report significant gender differences in the manifestation, course and recurrence of depressive disorder.[93,94] Also, large studies in primary care populations reported that women were significantly more depressed and functionally impaired than men but failed to point out other gender differences on symptom presentation. Further studies are still needed to clarify gender differences in the presentation of major depression.[95]

A challenge in assessment is to determine the primary nature of depressive symptoms in the context of active alcohol abuse or dependence. Depressive symptoms vary among individual patients in terms of specific symptoms, effects on alcohol use and effects on functioning. Depressive symptoms improve or remit after alcohol detoxification or several weeks of abstinence for some patients, but persist for others.[96]

Patients may be screened for depression at initial evaluation and again at the end of alcohol detoxification using one of the rating instruments. The persistence and severity of depressive symptoms can be more fully assessed using the Hamilton Rating Scale for Depression.[97] In addition, brief pen and paper questionnaires such as the Beck Depression Inventory (BDI) help the clinician and patient track changes in depressive symptoms over time.[98]

Major depressive disorder

- Single episode
- Recurrent

Dysthymic disorder

Depressive disorder not otherwise specified

Table 8
DSM-IV depressive disorders

- Depressed mood for 2 weeks

- Markedly diminished interest or pleasure in all, or almost all, activities

- Significant weight loss when not dieting or weight gain (e.g. a change of more than 5% of body weight in a month), or decrease or increase in appetite

- Insomnia or hypersomnia

- Psychomotor agitation or retardation

- Fatigue or loss of energy

- Feelings of worthlessness or excessive or inappropriate guilt

- Diminished ability to think or concentrate, or indecisiveness

- Recurrent thoughts of death, recurrent suicidal ideation without a specific plan, or a suicide attempt or a specific plan for committing suicide

Table 9
DSM-IV symptoms of major depression

> **Depressed mood for at least 2 years**
>
> **Presence, while depressed, of two (or more) of the following**
>
> - Poor appetite or overeating
> - Insomnia or hypersomnia
> - Low energy or fatigue
> - Low self-esteem
> - Poor concentration or difficulty making decisions
> - Feelings of hopelessness

Table 10
DSM-IV criteria for dysthymic disorder

Diagnostic issues

Alcohol-induced depressive symptoms usually improve within 3 weeks of abstinence.[99] However, determining whether depressive symptoms in a patient with alcohol dependence are caused by the use of alcohol or are part of the depressive disorder can be difficult. Alcohol can mask, cause or exacerbate depression. Alcohol use can induce depressive symptoms during an intoxication or withdrawal state, or as a result of persistent and chronic heavy use.[96] The high frequency of additional psychiatric disorders, such as attention deficit disorder-residual type and personality disorders such as antisocial, narcissistic or borderline personality disorder, also complicate assessment. Although there are no specific diagnostic tests for depression, the following clinical observations may help in establishing the diagnosis.

Temporal relationship

- Onset of depression prior to alcohol abuse problem
- Depressive symptoms persisted through prolonged period of abstinence
- In recently abstinent patients with alcohol dependence, depressive symptoms persisted beyond 2–4 weeks of abstinence

Phenomenological presentation

- Severity of depressive symptoms disproportionate to severity of alcohol use
- The presence of severe indicators of suicidal risk
- Symptoms not typically associated with the type of substance or the dose used (e.g. severe delusional depression)

The presence of other indicators of primary depressive disorder

- Family history of depression

Table 11
Clinical guidelines that help distinguish primary depression from alcohol-induced depression

Unless there has been a clear prior documentation of a primary major depressive disorder, such diagnosis should be withheld if a person is intoxicated or in a drug withdrawal state, given that most symptoms of depressive disorder may also be produced by alcoholism.

An alcohol-free observation period allows for close monitoring and ensures a drug- or alcohol-free state, and is very helpful in establishing the diagnosis. When available, an integrated treatment programme that can focus on both the alcoholism and depression should be used. Although opinions differ as to the *length* of the alcohol-free period during which an individual should be observed before establishing a primary psychiatric diagnosis, recent evidence indicates that depressive symptoms change little in patients with depression and alcoholism subsequent to 1 week of being alcohol free.[100,101] This is in contrast to the 4-week alcohol-free observation suggested by DSM-IV.[62]

Considering the temporal relationship between the appearance of symptoms and alcohol use may also aid in the diagnostic process. Depressed symptoms that occurred before the patient used alcohol, or symptoms that occurred during long periods of abstinence, are likely to indicate a primary depressive disorder.

Finally, obtaining a careful history of prior psychiatric illness may reveal clear past episodes of depression. Such episodes can be particularly useful in clarifying diagnostic questions if they occurred during a period of abstinence from substance abuse. Also, the presence of a family history of depressive illness may point to the likelihood of primary depressive illness.

Assessment of violent and aggressive behaviour

Suicide

Given the very high risk of suicidal behaviour and completed suicide among these patients, the clinician needs to evaluate: (1) current suicidal ideation, plan and intent; (2) the circumstance, severity and lethality of any suicidal gesture or attempt; (3) the availability of suicide method; and (4) the presence of risk factors for suicide.[102] The likelihood of suicide increases as the number of risk factors increases in the same individual. The presence of four suicide risk factors helped identify 80% of those at highest risk for suicide. Alcohol patients are especially at risk of committing impulsive suicidal acts while intoxicated, or during 'a blackout' state.[31,51] Drinking prior to suicide completion was found in almost all of completed suicides.[102]

- Recent heavy drinking
- Talk or threat of suicide
- Little social support
- Unemployment
- Living alone
- Serious medical problem

Table 12
Risk factors for suicide

Violence

Since male depressed patients with alcohol dependence are at increased risk for violent and aggressive behaviour, violence should be assessed during the evaluation. Violent behaviour can occur as part of alcohol intoxication or as a manifestation of associated psychopathology, such as depressive agitated state, antisocial personality disorder or agitated withdrawal delirium.

Assessment of the risk of violence includes a review of the history of past violence, drug abuse, threats to specific people and the availability of weapons. The presence of impaired impulse control, coping ability with aggressive urges, the degree of therapeutic alliance, the ability to contract for safety, and compliance with medications and treatment should also be carefully examined.[103]

- Schizophrenia; paranoid type
- Bipolar disorder, manic, mixed and depressed states
- Major depression with or without psychotic features
- Intermittent explosive disorder
- Post-traumatic stress disorder
- Cluster B personality disorders: especially antisocial, borderline and narcissistic personality disorders
- Other substance use, especially stimulant intoxication, hallucinogens, phencyclidine, inhalants and other depressants
- Conduct disorders and attention deficit disorders
- Delirium, dementia, mental retardation and seizure disorders

Table 13
Comorbid psychiatric diagnoses that may increase risk of violence

Getting the patient to accept help

Common barriers in seeking treatment

While some patients willingly accept recommendations to seek treatment for a mood disorder, alcohol use disorder or problems with violence, many do not despite the serious nature of their problems. They refuse treatment recommendations, accept them but then fail to actually follow through with the treatment referral, drop out of treatment prematurely or comply poorly with the actual treatment plan. For example, they may miss treatment sessions, fail to take medications as prescribed or not follow other specific recommendations made by the treating professional. Resistance is common so the caregiver should focus on understanding factors affecting motivation of the patient to engage in treatment and ways in which resistance can be lowered so that the patient follows through with the treatment referral.

Chart 1 summarizes the major factors affecting adherence to the recommendations of a professional to get help for depression, alcoholism or violence. These include client-, illness- or symptom-related factors, relationship and social support variables, and treatment and system variables.

It is usually a combination of factors that impact adversely on a patient's willingness to engage in treatment. Awareness of these common internal and external barriers in seeking help can help the clinician develop strategies to increase the chances that a patient will engage in treatment.

How to facilitate referrals to specialized treatment programmes

There are a number of strategies that the physician or other health care professional can use to increase the odds of a patient following through with specific recommendations for treatment of the problem of depression, alcoholism or violence. Chart 2 summarizes clinical strategies and Chart 3 summarizes systems strategies that can improve the patient's adherence with the treatment referral and ongoing participation.

Patients with alcohol use disorders and problems with violence often deny or minimize their problems, or the adverse effects of these problems on their lives or the lives of others such as family members. As a result, they may believe they do not need any treatment. Or, they may believe that they can change on their own without the help of others. By using motivational enhancement strategies,[104] the clinician can increase the likelihood that the patient will follow through with the recommendations to seek specialized help. These strategies have been used successfully with a variety of problems including alcohol use disorders,[105,106] opiate addiction,[107] obese women with diabetes,[108] patients with the dual disorders of substance abuse and depressive illness,[109-111] and patients with psychotic disorders.[112] These approaches utilize the strategies of 'Motivational Interviewing' as developed by Miller and Rollnick,[113] which aim to increase patients' readiness for treatment and motivation to change. Rather than see motivation as a 'trait' of the patient, this approach views motivation as a 'state' that can be affected by the clinician. Low motivation is seen as

Client variables	Illness- and symptom-related variables	Relationship and social support variables	Treatment and system variables
• Motivation • Beliefs • Stigma • Expectations • Satisfaction with treatment • Personality • Other addictions or compulsions (gambling, smoking, etc.) • Other life events or problems	• Symptoms of addiction • Symptoms of psychiatric illness • Obsessions or cravings to use • Social anxiety • Previous history of illness and relapse • Failure to catch early warning signs of relapse • Improvement in symptoms or problems	• Negative social supports • Unstable living situation • Poverty • Homelessness	• Therapeutic alliance • Friendliness of treatment staff • Competence of staff • Demands on counsellor • Supervision of staff • Access to treatment evaluation • Characteristics of treatment setting • Type of treatment offered and choices available • Duration of treatment regimen • Intensity of treatment programme • Appropriateness of treatment recommendations • Medication-related problems • Expense and accessibility of treatment • Ineffective or minimally effective treatment • Continuity of care • Availability of other services • Staff morale • Agency's fiscal health

Adapted from Daley DC, Zuckoff A. *Improving Treatment Compliance: Counseling and Systems Strategies for Substance Abuse and Dual Disorders.* Hazelden: Center City, MN; 1999, 40.[110]

Chart 1
Factors affecting compliance

a clinical problem to be addressed and resolved rather than as a reason not to engage the patient in treatment.

Therapeutic relationship
- Express empathy and concern
- Convey helpfulness in attitudes and behaviours
- Encourage discussions of the counselling process
- Encourage discussions of client–counsellor relationship

Motivation
- Accept ambivalence as normal
- Accept and appreciate small changes
- Accept varying levels of readiness to change
- Anticipate non-compliance at various stages of treatment
- Discuss prior history of compliance
- Discuss current compliance problems immediately

Treatment preparation
- Provide aftercare counselling prior to discharge from residential or inpatient care
- Help the client anticipate roadblocks to change
- Explore expectations and hopes for treatment

Treatment plan development
- Negotiate rather than dictate change plans
- Emphasize responsibility to the client
- Regularly review treatment goals and progress
- Discuss pros and cons of treatment
- Discuss pros and cons of self-help groups
- Discuss pros and cons of abstinence
- Provide options regarding treatment

Continued

Chart 2
Counselling strategies to improve adherence

Treatment process and strategies
- Provide interventions based on empirical support
- Change treatment frequency and intensity as needed
- Provide direct feedback to client
- Discuss client's reaction to feedback
- Provide reinforcement for treatment compliance
- Provide reinforcement for compliance with abstinence
- Address social anxiety about treatment groups or self-help groups

Family involvement
- Provide education to the client and family
- Elicit family support and involvement
- Address questions and concerns of the family

Symptom monitoring: psychiatric disorders
- Monitor psychiatric symptoms
- Address persistent or residual psychiatric symptoms
- Monitor psychiatric relapse warning signs

Symptom monitoring: substance use disorders
- Monitor substance use recovery issues
- Monitor cravings and thoughts of using substances
- Monitor people, places, events and close calls
- Focus on client's motivation
- Monitor substance use relapse warning signs

Medications
- Address medication issues
- Prepare client for taking medications
- Monitor medication compliance
- Address adverse side effects of lack of efficacy of medications
- Facilitate medication changes for ineffective medicines
- Facilitate augmentation therapy
- Prepare for negative reactions to medications from family or self-help group members

Adapted from Daley, DC Zuckoff A. *Improving Treatment Compliance: Counseling and Systems Strategies for Substance Abuse and Dual Disorders.* Center City, MN; Hazelden, 1999, 83.[110]

- Develop a clinic philosophy on compliance
- Encourage staff training on motivational and compliance counselling
- Provide easy access to treatment
- Offer flexible appointment times
- Offer consistent appointment times
- Call and remind clients of the initial evaluation session
- Call clients who fail to show for the initial evaluation
- Call clients or family members prior to regularly scheduled treatment sessions
- Use prompts to remind clients of scheduled sessions
- Use written compliance contracts
- Use creative ways of scheduling treatment appointments
- Outreach to poorly compliant clients
- Encourage treatment drop outs to return for services
- Determine the reasons for poor compliance or early treatment drop out
- Use case management services
- Help the client access other services
- Contact client to make sure referrals were followed up
- Provide assistance with practical problems
- Establish clinic and counsellor thresholds for acceptable levels of treatment compliance or completion
- Conduct regular client and family satisfaction surveys
- Continuously seek quality improvement
- Offer integrated treatment for clients with dual disorders

Adapted from Daley DC, Zuckoff A. *Improving Treatment Compliance: Counseling and Systems Strategies for Substance Abuse and Dual Disorders.* Center City, MN; Hazelden, 1999, 83.[110]

Chart 3
System strategies to improve compliance

While more extensive information is available elsewhere describing the theory underlying motivational approaches and clinical interventions,[104,110,113,114] the key components are summarized in the acronym FRAMES.

- **Feedback**: the physician or other caregiver provides the patient with specific feedback about diagnosis or problems assessed through clinical interviews, medical records, laboratory reports and/or collateral data (e.g. from a family member). This feedback gives the patient valuable information about the diagnoses, effects of the problem(s), possible interactions among several problems (e.g. violence and alcohol dependence or depression and alcohol abuse) that may lead to agreeing to accept a referral for specialized treatment. For example, we conducted a psychiatric evaluation on a fireman who presented with the chief complaint of depression. He was diagnosed with both major depression, single episode and alcohol dependence. We gave him specific feedback on these diagnoses with the recommendation that he become involved in outpatient treatment in a dual diagnosis programme that could address both of his disorders. He reluctantly accepted this recommendation and engaged in outpatient psychotherapy and then later agreed to take an antidepressant. Feedback was used initially to help him make a decision to accept ongoing treatment, and was used later to help him agree to take antidepressants since his depression improved only moderately despite continued abstinence from alcohol. With alcohol problems, feedback can incorporate any significant laboratory findings (e.g. high blood alcohol levels, elevated liver enzymes, related medical disorders that are caused or exacerbated by alcohol abuse), withdrawal symptoms, changes in tolerance to alcohol, and behaviours or problems associated with the alcohol use (e.g. family, legal, work). When the patient with an alcohol problem also evidences a clinical depression and/or problem with violence, feedback can incorporate information about these problems too.

- **R**esponsibility: the physician stresses that the decision to seek help or change is the sole responsibility of the patient. While recommendations can be provided about specific problems and possible treatment strategies, ultimately the patient must bear the responsibility for the disorders or problems, and the decision to engage in treatment. Specific and concrete feedback regarding diagnoses and problems caused by the patient's alcohol use, violence or depression may instil guilt and motivate the patient to seek help.

- **A**dvice: the patient is given specific advice on how to deal with the problem. For example, the physician might say to the patient who has problem with violence 'We've seen other people like yourself who've had trouble controlling their anger or becoming violent really benefit from therapy. I'd strongly advise you to get help and would like to recommend that you see Dr Johnson....'. Or 'You told me you're worried about your drinking and how it's affecting your health and family. I would recommend you stop drinking altogether since there's a good chance your liver would return to normal and you can work out your problems with your wife. I think you would gain a lot by getting involved in treatment at...'

- **M**enu: different treatment or change options are provided to the patient who chooses from among them. The physician might say to a moderately depressed patient 'I can refer you to the Bellefield clinic that offers several different treatment programmes for depression or to Dr Howell's practice. Either of these programmes can provide you with therapy and medications if needed.' Or, a patient with alcohol dependence may be told 'Many of our other patients with alcohol problems have benefited from professional treatment. Let me tell you about several of these programmes and you can decide which one you would like to attend.'

- **E**mpathy: a positive therapeutic alliance or relationship with a patient is built on empathy, or the ability to accept, understand and have a sincere desire to help the patient. While it is easy to take an empathetic stance with a depressed patient, it often is more difficult to feel empathy towards the patient with an alcohol and/or violence problem. Judgemental and negative attitudes or reactions will impede the ability to help these patients, so the physician or caregiver must be aware of personal attitudes, perceptions and beliefs regarding these types of problems. If, for example, alcohol dependence is viewed as bad behaviour and a flaw in the individual rather than a serious biopsychosocial disorder, the professional will be less able to help the affected patient.

- **S**elf-efficacy: the caregiver supports the patient's belief in the ability to make positive changes whenever possible, and increase a sense of optimism that things can get better. For example, the patient may be told 'It sounds like you've succeeded in the past coping with your depression when you had the support of your wife and saw a therapist. You're in a good position to do this again, which I think will help your depression.' Or, 'You've been very honest about how much rage you feel and how close you came to hitting your wife and kids. The fact that you walked away and took time out was good. While it's been hard, you have managed to control your violent impulses. Let's talk more about other things that can help you stay in control so no one gets hurt.'

Introduction

Treatment of dual diagnosis patients has been conceptualized into several phases:[3] (1) an acute phase focused on treatment engagement, detoxification from drug and/or alcohol and stabilization of the depressive illness; (2) a continuation phase focused on further treatment of symptoms, and making personal and lifestyle changes; and (3) a maintenance phase focused on reducing the risk of relapse. This is best accomplished in a treatment programme that can address all of the patient's disorders and problems.

Integrated pharmacotherapy with psychotherapeutic interventions

Pharmacotherapy is most effective when combined with therapy, counselling and/or self-help programme attendance. Given the chronic nature of the depression and alcoholism, the high frequency of violence, other psychiatric and drug use disorders, and the multiplicity of psychosocial difficulties, a team approach and a therapeutic milieu is necessary for many patients. A therapeutic milieu refers to a structured, intensive, group-oriented treatment programme in a residential or non-residential setting. Patients receive support and feedback from each other in addition to the professional team members. A major role of therapy, in addition to addressing recovery issues for alcoholism and depressive disorder or violence, is to enhance medication compliance.

Facilitating medication acceptance and compliance

Antidepressant medications improve depressive symptoms of alcoholics, whether due to primary or secondary depression.[100,101,115] However, patients may deny, minimize or have misconceptions regarding the severity of the disorders as well as the need for treatment, including medications. Patient education about medications, side effects and potential adverse interactions with alcohol or illicit drugs, as well as the education of physicians, other health providers and self-help programmes about this dual diagnosis condition, are essential in overcoming these impediments.[116]

Patient-related factors

- Denial, minimization, poor compliance
- Erroneous expectations and misunderstanding of the role of medications

Environmental factors

- Family or self-help group members' misconception regarding the use of 'mood altering' drugs

Physician or caregiver factors

- Fear that medications are unnecessary because the psychiatric symptoms are drug induced
- Fear of toxic interaction with drugs or alcohol
- Lack of efficacy if drug abuse is active
- Fear of 'enabling' the patient
- Fear of being manipulated by the patient

Table 14
Impediments to antidepressant use

Furthermore, several general treatment issues regarding medication use in depressed patients with alcoholism are important to observe, especially during the early stabilization phase of treatment.[117]

- Ascertain the diagnosis
- Prescribe medications with low abuse potential (e.g. avoid narcotics or benzodiazepines)
- Prescribe medications that have low lethality on overdose (e.g. SRIs)
- Dispense limited amount
- Maintain frequent contact and closely monitor medication side effects and treatment compliance
- Encourage initial involvement with a structured, intensive treatment programme (e.g. several meetings per week)
- Educate patient on medication effects, side effects and expected response
- Discuss patient's attitude, thoughts and feelings regarding medication
- Prepare the patient for the possibility of getting pressure from self-help group members to stop taking medications
- Perform random urine or plasma toxicology screens

Table 15
Prescribing medications in the context of alcohol or drug abuse

Pharmacological treatment of alcohol withdrawal in depressed patients with alcohol dependence

The major goals of detoxification are to prevent or reduce withdrawal symptoms, prevent withdrawal complications, and persuade the patient to get involved in treatment and an ongoing programme of recovery.[88] Benzodiazepines are the medications of choice for treating alcohol withdrawal.[118] Most frequently used agents include long-acting compounds such as diazepam and chlordiazepoxide, and intermediate-acting compounds such as lorazepam, oxazepam and temazepam.[117] The pharmacokinetic profile of the long-acting diazepam and chlordiaxepoxide, and their active metabolites, provide improved control over the withdrawal symptoms.[119] Intermediate-acting benzodi-azepines, especially those without active metabolites, are particularly useful in patients with compromised liver functions.

An enhanced method for the management of alcohol withdrawal is the introduction of objective assessment scales to guide medication administration, coupled with the use of the diazepam loading dose. This method appears to be superior to the traditional method of alcohol detoxification. This procedure allows for frequent and more reliable assessment of the progression of the withdrawal syndrome, thus preventing the development of either withdrawal complications or side effects caused by excessive medication dose.[119] We have used this procedure successfully in a large group of comorbid psychiatric and alcohol-dependent patients, most of whom had major depression.[88]

Pharmacotherapeutic approaches in depressed patients with alcohol dependence

When to initiate antidepressant medication

As depressive symptoms improve significantly subsequent to alcohol detoxification, a primary question that faces the physician is to determine the need for antidepressant medications. Clinical trials of depressed patients with alcohol dependence have reported only modest improvements in depressive symptoms beyond the first week of detoxification for patients who were randomized to placebo.[100,101,115] The DSM-IV guidelines for determining the presence of primary versus secondary depression within the context of alcohol use disorders extends this period up to 4 weeks.[120] Other studies report that 3 weeks may be required before alcohol-induced depression clears.[99] The decision to initiate antidepressant medications should be weighed for the individual patient in terms of benefits versus risks of withholding antidepressant medications.

Two main approaches to the pharmacotherapy of comorbid depression and alcoholism have been advanced. A monotherapy approach, where the major depression component is treated with an antidepressant medication. Improved alcohol outcome is also expected with a good response to the antidepressant medication. A more recent approach is to combine antidepressants with medications such as naltrexone hydrochloride that are used to decrease the desire to drink alcohol.[121,122]

Antidepressant monotherapy for depressed patients with alcohol dependence

Although the primary goal is to stabilize the depressive disorder, antidepressants often also reduce alcohol use. There are reports of good prognostic outcomes for the alcohol use among depressed alcoholic females[123] but not males. Moreover, several newer antidepressant medications such as the serotonin reuptake inhibitors (SRIs) may possess intrinsic therapeutic effects on moderating alcohol use. Serotonin appears to play a major role in the alcohol reinforcing effect.[124] There is an inverse relationship between serotonin levels in the central nervous system and alcohol consumption in humans and animals. Diverse subtypes of serotonin receptors appear to be involved in the reinforcing effect of alcohol. Enhancement of these receptors by the use of SRIs usually leads to decreased alcohol consumption.[125] The serotonergic system is also believed to influence the compulsive consumatory behaviour related to the addictive use of substance in particular.[126] SRIs decrease the craving for alcohol and also have an indirect effect on alcohol consumption by alleviating the anxiety and depressive symptoms which in turn have been implicated in stress reaction and compulsory drinking.[127]

Clinical trials in depressed patients with alcohol dependence

A limited number of studies addressed the efficacy of antidepressant monotherapy in depressed patients with alcohol dependence. Studies evaluating the tricyclic antidepressants imipramine and desipramine reported efficacy for these compounds in treating the depression of those with alcohol dependence but had inconsistent efficacy in treating the excessive alcohol use of these patients.[101,115] Imipramine was not found effective in treating excessive drinking, while desipramine was found to decrease both excessive drinking and the secondary depression of the alcohol dependent.

SRIs, on the other hand, are useful in decreasing both the depressive symptoms and excessive drinking in patients with alcohol dependence. Cornelius et al.[100] have shown that fluoxetine is helpful in decreasing the alcohol use as well as the depressive symptoms compared to placebo in the severely depressed alcohol dependent. The fluoxetine group consumed less alcohol and stayed sober longer than the placebo group. These patients had a greater decrease in their depressive symptoms than the placebo group.

Selecting an antidepressant medication

There are increasingly more pharmacological choices available for the treatment of depressive disorders. The depressed alcohol dependent represent a significant subgroup with special characteristics and vulnerabilities. Therefore, a choice of medication should be largely dictated by these needs. For example, chronic alcohol use induces the hepatic enzyme system into accelerating the metabolism of the tricyclic antidepressants.[28,128] On the other hand, acute alcohol intoxication may significantly impair liver metabolism of the tricyclic antidepressants, especially amitriptyline and imipramine, resulting in a substantial increase in the blood levels of these compounds.

- Effective for both disorders
- Has favourable side effect profile
- Has low potential for abuse
- Does not produce dependence
- Does not enhance the CNS effects of alcohol or other abused drugs
- Has low lethality potential on overdose
- Has low potential for adverse interactions with drugs or alcohol
- Has beneficial effects on aggression and violent behaviour
- Has beneficial effects on sleep, anxiety and impulse control symptoms

Table 16
Desirability profile of antidepressants for depressed alcoholics

Currently, published studies testing the efficacy of antidepressants in comorbid major depression and alcohol dependence have only included fluoxetine, desipramine and imipramine. Citalopram, on the other hand, has been tested in patients with alcohol dependence but without major depression.[129,130] The citalopram 40 mg dose, but not the 20 mg, was found to decrease alcohol use in an earlier double-blind cross-over study.[129] In a subsequent double-blind placebo-controlled study, citalopram 40 mg was found to decrease alcohol consumption more than placebo during the first week of treatment, although effects on alcohol consumption were not different from placebo at 12 weeks (study termination).[130] It is not clear if this temporal difference in efficacy reflects a loss of drug effect or if it is an artefact of differential attrition. Specifically, patients who are not doing well commonly drop out of placebo-controlled studies long before the 12-week follow-up. The authors of that study speculate, however, that tolerance to the effect of citalopram through some neurobiological adaptive changes may have developed. However, in addition to the efficacy, safety and tolerability profile, useful antidepressants would also possess therapeutic effects for depressive symptoms, such as impulsivity, anxiety and sleep difficulties that are common among depressed patients with alcohol dependence. Studies have shown that these symptoms have important prognostic significance. Comorbid anxiety symptoms have been linked to high frequency of suicidal behaviour among depressed patients.[131] Sleep difficulties appear to be an important prognostic indicator for reoccurrence of depressive disorder[132] as well as relapse to alcohol use.[133]

Following are the most widely used antidepressants compared on the suggested desirability profile.

	Citalopram	Fluoxetine	Fluvoxamine	Paroxetine	Sertraline
Compliance/ tolerance	High	High	High	High	High
Abuse/ dependence potential	No	No	No	No	No
CNS potentiation of alcohol	No	No	No	No	No
Effective for depression	Yes	Yes	Yes	Yes	Yes
Effective for alcoholism in depressed patients	Not tested*	Yes	Not tested	Not tested	Possible
Lethality potential	Low	Low	Low	Low	Low
Alcohol metabolism interactions	No	No	No	No	No

Table 17
Serotonin reuptake inhibitors (SRIs)
* Tested patients with alcohol dependence without comorbid major depression[129,130]

	Mirtazapine	Venlafaxine	Nefazodone	Bupropion	Trazodone
Compliance/ tolerance	High	Moderate	Moderate	Moderate	High
Abuse/ dependence potential	No	No	No	No	No
CNS potentiation of alcohol	Yes	No	↑Sedation	No	↑Sedation
Effective for depression	Yes	Yes	Yes	Yes	Questionable
Effective for alcoholism in depressed patients	Not tested	Not tested	Not tested	Not tested	Not tested
Lethality potential	Low	Low	Low	Moderate to high	Moderate to high
Alcohol metabolism interactions	Low	No	Low	No	Low

Table 18
Non-classic SRI antidepressants

	Tricyclics	MAOIs
Compliance/tolerance	Low	Low
Abuse/dependence potential	Possible	Possible
CNS potentiation of alcohol	High	High
Effective for depression	Yes	Yes
Effective for alcoholism in depressed patients	Questionable	Not tested
Lethality potential	Very high	Very high
Alcohol metabolism interactions	High	High

Table 19
Tricyclics and MAO inhibitors

Combined medication approach

This approach capitalizes on the different neurochemical profile of the medications that affect different neurotransmitter systems involved in alcoholism and depression. A hypothesized additive or synergistic therapeutic effect may result from the combined medications. A useful combination is that of an SRI with an opiate antagonist, such as the combination of fluoxetine, sertraline or citalopram with naltrexone.[122] Fluoxetine targets the depressive symptoms, while naltrexone targets alcohol use. Both naltrexone and fluoxetine may also reduce excessive alcohol use. While there are no published double-blind clinical trials evaluating the efficacy of such combination, our open-label study of the depressed alcohol dependent who are resistant to SRIs alone reported a significant decrease in excessive alcohol use and improvement in depressive symptoms.[121] Furthermore, this combination was well tolerated by patients and the addition of naltrexone did not alter fluoxetine or norfluoxetine blood concentrations for most patients.[134]

Pharmacotherapy of alcoholism

Pharmacological agents currently available to treat alcoholism include: (1) aversive agents such as disulfiram; (2) the opioid antagonist naltrexone hydrochloride; and (3) the GABA analogue acamprosate (available in many European countries).[135,136]

Although disulfiram may be useful in a subgroup of select patients,[137,138] its side effect profile and potential extensive interaction with other medications may limit its usefulness in depressed male patients with alcohol dependence, especially those with other psychiatric or medical comorbidity and those with poor impulse control.[139] Naltrexone appears to be safe in combination with antidepressant medications, especially of the SRI class.[121,140] Acamprosate has a favourable side effect profile and has no interactions with alcohol as it is eliminated unchanged through the kidneys and it may prove very useful in dual diagnosis patients.

- Aversive agent
- Irreversible inhibition of the enzyme aldehyde dehydrogenase
- Accumulation of acetaldehyde causes the acetaldehyde syndrome or disulfiram–ethanol reaction
- Dose range 125–250 mg/day
- Problematic side effect profile with liver toxicity and neuropathy
- Generalized enzyme inhibitors
- Liver toxicity monitoring is essential
- May precipitate psychopathology including psychosis or depression
- Contraindicated in severely ill patients
- May be used in mild non-psychotic depressive or anxiety disorders
- Multiple medication/medication interactions

Table 20
Disulfiram

- Pure opiate antagonist
- Decreases alcohol use and alcohol relapse probably by influencing the positive reinforcing effects of alcohol
- Dose range 50–100 mg/day
- Appears safe mixed with alcohol
- Limited side effects profile mostly nausea and anxiety
- Reported liver damage at higher dosage
- Precipitates severe opiate withdrawal
- Blocks the effects of opiate analgesia
- Does not worsen depression
- Well tolerated in combination with antidepressants

Table 21
Naltrexone hydrochloride

- Decreases alcohol use probably by influencing the negative reinforcing effects of alcohol
- Current dose is 2000 mg/day
- Does not interact with alcohol
- Well tolerated
- Side effects limited to itching and soft stool/diarrhoea
- Not addictive
- Not metabolized by the liver
- Excreted unchanged through the kidneys
- No reported experience with dual diagnosis

Table 22
Acamprosate

Pharmacotherapy of violence

Pharmacological agents used to treat violent behaviour target one or more of the neurobiological mechanisms underlying aggression and violence. These include the serotonergic, noradrenergic, GABAergic, dopaminergic system and the anti-androgen drug medroxyprogesterone. Serotonergic system dysfunction has been the most widely studied and linked to the aetiology of violent, aggressive and impulsive behaviour. These abnormalities are especially prominent in early-onset alcoholism.[141]

Antidepressants	Anxiolytics
• Serotonin reuptake inhibitors	• Buspirone
	• Benzodiazepines
Mood stabilizers	
	Others
• Lithium carbonate	
• Valproic acid	• Beta-blockers
• Carbamazepine	• Stimulants
	• Medroxyprogesterone acetate
Antipsychotics	
• Classic neuroleptic agents	
• Atypical antipsychotics	

Table 23

Pharmacotherapeutic agents used to treat violent behaviour

Serotonin reuptake inhibitors have been found to be useful in reducing aggression in a variety of psychiatric disorders including depression,[142] obsessive–compulsive disorder,[143] autism,[144] mental retardation[145] and schizophrenia.[146] Vartiainen et al. found that citalopram reduced aggression in a group of chronically violent patients with schizophrenia.[146]

Mood stabilizers have also been used extensively to treat aggressive behaviour among psychiatric patients. Lithium carbonate appears to be helpful in a variety of situations.[147–149] Lithium increases brain serotonin functions[150] and it may also enhance the effects of serotonin reuptake inhibitors. Anticonvulsant mood stabilizers such as carbamazepine and valproic acid are specially useful in reducing aggression in patients with abnormal electroencephalogram and temporal lobe epilepsy, as well as in patients with intermittent explosive disorders.[8]

The anti-anxiety drug buspirone, a serotonergic agent, has shown some usefulness in the treatment of aggression.[151,152] Although benzodiazepines have been used to control violent and aggressive behaviour, their long-term use is not recommended for patients with alcohol dependence or other substance use disorders.

Newer or atypical antipsychotic medications, such as olanzapine and clozapine, may also be useful in controlling violent and aggressive behaviour.[153,154] Olanzapine may be particularly useful given its broad spectrum of action and tolerability.[155–157]

Psychotherapies

A number of brief psychotherapy and counselling approaches have been shown to be effective with alcohol use disorders with no one treatment showing superiority over the others. The more common manually driven treatments include Motivational Enhancement Therapy (MET),[104,113] Cognitive–Behavioural or Social Skills therapies (CB)[158] and Twelve-Step Facilitation Therapy (TSF).[159] A recent major study comparing MET, CB and TSF found no significant differences in outcome between the three treatments, but found all treatments to have a significant positive effect at 1 year follow-up on reducing the percentage of days drinking (80% pre-treatment to 20% post-treatment) and number of drinks per day (17 per day at pre-treatment to 3 at post-treatment follow-up). These treatments involved 6–12 individual treatment sessions over several months. Several marital and family treatments have been found to be effective in helping patients with alcohol problems enter, comply and complete treatment, and in helping stabilize marital or family relationships.[160–164] More recent family work has focused on strategies to help the family get the alcohol impaired member into treatment.[165]

Two psychotherapies effective in the treatment of depression include Interpersonal Therapy (IP)[166] and Cognitive–Behavioral Therapy (CBT).[167] These treatments involve up to 20 individual sessions over a period of several months. IP focuses on helping the patient reduce depression by resolving grief, addressing interpersonal disputes, life changes or major role transitions, and/or interpersonal deficits. CBT focuses on helping the patient identify, challenge and modify cognitive distortions that contribute to depression. CBT also focuses on helping the patient change specific behaviours such as becoming more assertive in interpersonal situations, structuring time and building pleasant activities into one's day.

Violent behaviour is frequently associated with alcohol use disorders, mood disorders, psychotic disorders, impulse control disorders, sexual offences and deviance, and anti-social and borderline personality disorders. Treatment of the violence is often incorporated into the overall treatment of the disorders. For example, CBT has been adapted by Freeman, Beck and others[168] for use with personality disorders, some of which include violent behaviours as one of the problems or symptoms. Strategies such as helping the patient understand and change core beliefs related to violence and interpersonal relationships, and change problematic behaviours are part of CBT. In addition, the Dialectic Behavioral Therapy (DBT) model developed by Linehan[169,170] for the treatment of borderline personality disorder teaches a variety of 'skills' that can help the patient reduce and control violent behaviour. The DBT treatment programme involves a combination of individual and skill groups. Patients may also use medication for associated symptoms of psychosis, depression or mood lability. The overall general goal of DBT is to help the patient learn and refine skills in order to change behavioural, emotional and thinking patterns associated with problems that cause misery and distress for the patient. Specific goals relevant to the problem of violence include decreasing interpersonal chaos, labile emotions, negative mood states and impulsiveness, and focusing on increasing the skills of interpersonal effectiveness, emotion regulation and distress tolerance.[170] Each of these specific goals in turn focuses on a number of related goals such as reducing angry feelings or the inappropriate expression of it, reducing feelings of sadness and increasing the appropriate expression of it, and reducing other painful emotions. Each of these subgoals involves specific strategies for the patient to use such as increasing positive events, self-soothing the five senses, or distracting painful events or emotions with 'Wise Mind ACCEPTS' (Activities, Contributing, Comparisons, Emotions, Pushing away, Thoughts and Sensations).

Individual and group treatments utilizing cognitive, behavioural and relapse prevention strategies have also been integrated into residential and community-based 'treatment programmes' for a variety of sexual offences, some of which include elements of interpersonal violence.[171–173] In addition, there are other specialized treatment and recovery approaches for domestic abuse or violence,[174–176] rape and child molestation,[171] and sexual addiction.[177]

The treatment of patients with depression, alcoholism and/or violence problems involves the following strategies:

- Providing education to the patient and family regarding the disorder(s), the interaction among multiple disorders, the role of professional treatment including medications, the process of recovery, the process of relapse and the role of self-help programmes

- Helping the patient stabilize from acute symptoms of psychiatric illness (e.g. suicidality, homicidality, severe mood disturbance) and alcohol dependence (e.g. withdrawal symptoms), and to stop violence.

- Helping the patient increase motivation to change and participate in ongoing treatment and/or self-help programmes

- Helping the patient develop behavioural, cognitive and interpersonal coping skills to manage the mood disorder (e.g. persistent mood symptoms, depressive thinking or early signs of depression relapse), the alcohol use disorder (e.g. cravings to drink alcohol, social pressures to drink or early signs of relapse) or the violence problem (e.g. changing beliefs and thoughts about violence or retribution for perceived wrongs, identifying and managing triggers for rage or anger), and to make positive changes in self and/or lifestyle

- Involving the family or significant other in the treatment process

- Encouraging the patient to develop a recovery support system and become active in self-help groups

The specific treatment needs of a given patient, recommendations provided by the caregiver and response to actual treatment will depend on several variables. [22]

- Type and severity of mood disorder
- Type and severity of alcohol use disorder or other substance disorder
- Severity of violence problem and related psychiatric diagnoses
- Level of social anxiety (affects group treatment and self-help participation)
- Effects of disorder(s) on patient's functioning
- Effects of disorder(s) on patient's family
- Age, gender, employment status, ethnicity
- Level of acceptance of disorder(s) and motivation to change
- Personality
- Cognitive functioning
- Family and social supports
- Alliance with professional caregiver(s)
- Appropriateness of treatment regimen

Table 24
Factors mediating treatment needs and response

Continuum of care

Effective treatment of depression, alcoholism and/or violence may involve a number of different levels of care. Not all patients require the same level of care or same type of intervention. Cases in which a patient has multiple disorders should be referred to a programme or professional who can provide integrated treatment for the disorders. A depressed alcoholic is usually best treated in a programme that understands and can address both disorders. Too often, patients are treated adequately for one disorder while the other disorder is ignored or de-emphasized, which can lead to a poor response to treatment. While mental health or substance abuse treatment may be useful to patients in certain circumstances, patients with both types of disorders generally respond better to clinical approaches that provide an integrated focus on the disorders and related problems.

Multiple levels of care may be needed for the effective treatment of depression, alcoholism and/or violence. Patients may use only one level of care or move back and forth between levels of care, depending on their current problems and symptoms. In addition, programmes may be available for 'special populations' such as pregnant women, women with children, patients with persistent and chronic forms of mental illness including mood disorders, gay men and lesbians, multiple relapsers, or patients involved with the criminal justice system as a result of arrests for sexual offences, violent behaviours or other felonies. Regardless of their presenting problems or diagnoses, patients who have serious psychosocial problems such as being homeless, unemployed or without financial resources may benefit from the services of a case manager or social service agency. Finally, some patients will require medications to help treat the mood disorder, alcohol use disorder or violence problem (see 'Pharmacotherapy' chapter).

Acute care inpatient/ emergency	Short- or long-term residential	Ambulatory care
Psychiatric hospitalization	Psychiatric residential programmes	Partial hospital programme
Detoxification	Addiction rehabilitation programmes	Intensive outpatient programme
Dual diagnosis programmes	Therapeutic communities	Outpatient treatment programme
Brief stabilization programmes	Halfway houses	Aftercare programme
23 hour bed		

Table 25
The continuum of care for depression, alcoholism and violence

Psychosocial issues in recovery

The goals of treatment are to help patients stabilize from the major symptoms of their disorders, address problems contributing to or resulting from their disorders, learn to manage chronic conditions or programmes, and make specific intrapersonal or interpersonal changes. Involvement in professional treatment provides the patient with the opportunity to begin the process of recovery and make changes. The major issues in recovery that the patient may address relate to physical, behavioural, cognitive, family, interpersonal and social functioning, personal growth and lifestyle (Table 26). Specific areas of focus in therapy will depend on the motivation, and unique problems and needs of the patient.

Self-help programmes

Self-help programmes such as Alcoholics Anonymous (AA), Rational Recovery or SMART Recovery are commonly used with alcohol problems. Self-help programmes are also available for mood disorders and dual disorders. Problems with violence can sometimes be addressed within the context of these programmes. The caregiver can help the patient by providing education about self-help programmes, identifying and discussing patient resistances, questions or concerns regarding these programmes, examining how they may potentially help the patient with his or her specific disorders or problems, and facilitating entry into specific types of self-help groups. In some cases, it helps to have contacts in self-help programmes so that the patient can be called by other members of self-help groups or given names of specific individuals to call.

Physical/lifestyle

- Exercise
- Follow a healthy diet
- Rest and relaxation
- Take medications (if needed)
- Take care of medical problem
- Learn to structure time
- Engage in pleasant activities
- Achieve balance in life
- Engage in meditation

Psychological

- Monitor moods
- Manage negative moods
- Reduce anxiety
- Reduce boredom and emptiness
- Reduce guilt and shame
- Control anger/rage
- Address 'losses' (grief)

Personal growth/maintenance

- Address spirituality issues
- Develop relapse prevention plan for all disorders or problems
- Develop relapse interruption plan for all disorders or problems
- Use 'recovery tools' on ongoing basis

Behavioural/cognitive

- Accept the disorder(s) or problem(s)
- Control urges to drink alcohol or use drugs
- Change unhealthy beliefs and thoughts
- Reduce depressed thoughts
- Increase pleasant thoughts
- Reduce violent thoughts
- Control violent impulses
- Develop motivation to change
- Change self-defeating patterns of behaviour

Family/interpersonal/social

- Identify effects on family and significant relationships
- Involve family in treatment/recovery
- Resolve family/marital conflicts
- Make amends to family or other significant people harmed
- Manage high-risk people, places and events
- Engage in non-drinking activities or healthy leisure interests
- Address relationship or deficits
- Resist social pressures to drink alcohol
- Resolve work, school, financial, legal problems
- Learn to face versus avoid interpersonal conflicts
- Learn to ask for help and support
- Seek and use an AA sponsor

Table 26
Psychosocial issues in recovery

Alcoholism, depression and violence are chronic and relapsing problems for many patients.[178–180] While the ideal outcome of treatment is remission of symptoms of the disorders, early intervention in the relapse process can help limit adverse effects of a relapse. Depressed patients who stabilize from their acute symptoms and achieve a period of remission often require maintenance treatment in order to reduce the risk of future episodes. Other goals of the maintenance phase are to make personal and lifestyle changes to support recovery from all disorders, achieve social stability and deal with problems resulting from the disorders (e.g. family, vocational, economic).

Course of major depression

Approximately 30% of patients with major depression have only one lifetime episode, while the remaining have two or more with an expected five to six episodes throughout the lifetime;[181] 25% develop a chronic form of depressive illness.[182]

Over half of depressed patients relapse within 1 year after discontinuation of active medication. This rate increases to 74% by the second year and to 85% by the third year of discontinuation of medication. Maintenance antidepressant treatment substantially reduces the rate of recurrence of depression[183–185] and is recommended for patients who have had two episodes within the past 5 years or three lifetime episodes of depression.[186]

Several factors increase the risk of recurrent depression. These include an early age of onset of the first depressive episode, familial and genetic factors, comorbid psychopathology such as anxiety disorders, substance abuse, dysthymia, psychosis, depressive temperamental traits and personality disorders, and early exposure to environmental stressors.[178] A first depressive episode occurring after the age of 60 has also been considered a risk factor for recurrence. Furthermore, the number of prior episodes correlates with shorter periods of remission.[187,188] It has been proposed that repeated episodes accelerate the course of the illness with more frequent episodes occurring with shorter intervals of remission in between (e.g. the kindling hypothesis).[178,189]

A 15-year follow-up study found that 85% of the sample had a recurrent episode, with the mean and median time to recurrence occurring within 3 years of follow-up.[190] Predictors for recurrence included female gender, being single and having a longer duration of depression before the index episode.

Persistence of subsyndromal depressive symptoms is also a strong predictor of recurrence. The presence of subsyndromal symptoms in recovered individuals shortened the 'well time' threefold (68 versus 231 weeks).[190] Studies of depression in primary care settings also report high rates of relapse with subthreshold persistent symptoms among the predictors for relapse within 12 months. Other predictors include a history of two or more depressive episodes or chronic mood symptoms for 2 years.[191] Subjects with both risk factors were three times as likely to have a relapse and over half of them were likely to have subsequent relapse within a year.

Frank et al.[184] demonstrated that long-term antidepressant pharmacotherapy helps patients maintain a state of well-being. Indications for maintenance antidepressant therapy in depression include chronic depression, recurrent depression, severe and protracted episodes of depression, double depression (major depression and dysthymia), and residual dysthymia.[182]

Response	Significant reduction in depression symptoms below the threshold of a major depressive disorder diagnosis within the first 4 weeks of acute treatment.
Remission	Complete response of symptoms and return to baseline 'well' states, with no signs or symptoms of the illness. This is likely to occur within the first 12 weeks of acute treatment.
Recovery	If remission is sustained for up to 6–9 months then a recovery may be obtained.
Relapse	An exacerbation in depressive symptoms before a complete recovery has occurred.
Recurrence	A new depressive episode occurs after recovery.
Residual	The presence and persistence of subsyndromal depressive symptoms despite continued treatment and remission of the current episode.
Refractory	The persistence of the depressive episode despite adequate multiple treatment trials.

Table 27
Definitions of terms describing the course of depression (the 7 Rs)[178]

Alcohol effects on major depression

Alcohol use can lower the depressed patient's motivation with treatment and compliance with self-help participation, and adversely interfere with the pharmacokinetic and pharmacodynamic aspects of the antidepressant medications. Although many of the SRIs appear to be safe, even when alcohol has been consumed, these patients have other comorbid medical and psychiatric disorders that require other medications. This increases the likelihood of medication side effects and adverse interactions with alcohol, including the intensification of alcohol effects.

Alcohol-induced depression, anxiety and sleep symptoms contribute to recurrence of major depressive episodes. Sub-threshold depressive symptoms are among the strongest predictors of relapse and recurrence of depressive episodes. Alcohol use can also precipitate and potentiate suicidal or violent behaviours.

Alcohol use makes the stabilization of the depressive symptoms during the acute episode extremely difficult and it is one of the most common reasons for lack of response to medications. It contributes to the persistence of depressive symptoms during the continuation phase of treatment, increasing the chances for depressive relapse. Alcohol use also increases the chances for a reoccurrence of depressive episode in those who have fully recovered. Finally, kindling and sensitization mechanisms have been produced by repeated alcohol withdrawal in animal research and clinical studies of alcoholic populations. A kindling model has been advanced for recurrent major depression. It is unclear how these two models interact in patients with both recurrent major depression and alcohol dependence. It is likely that this process, which has prognostic significance, may be enhanced in depressed patients with alcohol dependence as compared to either those with non-alcohol recurrent major depression or to non-depressed patients with alcohol dependence.

Depression response	Interferes with response to medication, psychotherapy and compliance Worsens depressive symptoms
Depression remission	Prolongs the 'sick' state by maintaining symptoms and psychosocial stress
Depression recovery	Hampers recovery by maintaining persistent symptoms and impairing coping skills
Depression relapse	Increased risk for depression relapses
Depression recurrence	Increased likelihood of recurrences due to persistent subsyndromal symptoms, the kindling process and psychosocial stress

Table 28
Alcohol as a risk factor for major depression relapse and recurrence

Course of alcoholism

Alcoholism is a chronic, relapsing illness, which, in a substantial minority of cases may progress to a fatal outcome.[192] In the longest follow-up studies of two cohorts of patients with alcohol dependence, 18% of college students and 28% of an inner-city sample had died by the age of 60. Only 11% of the college student sample and 30% of the inner-city sample were abstinent. Relapse was rare only after maintaining sobriety for 5 years and a return to controlled drinking without eventual relapse was unlikely.[192]

Alcohol lapse and relapse

Many individuals with alcohol problems who quit for a period of time drink again at some point in their lives. Some lapse or have a single episode of use that does not lead to continued use and an eventual relapse in which drinking escalates. Others relapse or experience ongoing use of substances once they resume drinking. Lapses and relapses can vary from mild to severe in terms of quantity of alcohol used, duration of the drinking episode and adverse effects on the person's life. The greatest risk period during treatment or recovery for relapse is the first 3 months. Most lapses and relapses occur early because during this time patients are most likely to feel ambivalent about abstinence, have not developed a strong commitment to change or do not have the coping skills needed to meet the many demands and challenges of recovery (e.g. managing strong cravings, dealing with negative affect without drinking, using a support system). Although there are many commonalities across relapse situations, each patient needs an individualized plan that helps him or her anticipate and prepare for the possibility of relapse.

Causes of relapse

It is usually a combination of factors rather than one that contributes to alcohol relapse. For example, an alcohol-dependent person at a party may drink in response to pressures to drink alcohol from others only during times in which he or she feels anxious or bored. Drinking may be an attempt to reduce anxiety or boredom and to feel part of a group that is perceived to be having fun, or an alcohol-dependent person may drink mainly when upset and angry at a spouse following an argument because coping skills are lacking in managing interpersonal conflict. Therefore, it is not only the 'high-risk' situation that is a mediator of relapse but the alcohol-dependent person's ability to use coping skills to manage the situation. The following lists the most common factors contributing to relapse.[180]

• Negative emotional states	38%
• Social pressures	18%
• Interpersonal conflicts	18%
• Urges or temptations to drink	11%
• Positive emotional states	3%
• Other	12%

Table 29
Factors contributing to alcohol relapse

Major depression as a risk factor for alcohol relapse

Depression increases the vulnerability to alcohol relapse through its impact on the adaptational capacity of patients with alcohol dependence. Recent severe stressors as well as chronic difficulties that are highly threatening are associated with high risk of relapse.[193] Studies of abstinent patients with alcohol dependence indicate that stressors that increase the risk of addiction relapse are those that exceed the personal adaptation capacity of the individual.[194] Depression mediates the effect of stress on alcohol relapse.[195] Depressive disorders impact negatively on all areas identified by Brown et al.[194] as predictive of relapse in abstinent patients with alcohol dependence experiencing stress. Depressive disorder can cause severe impairment in coping skills and self-efficacy through a host of neurovegetative and cognitive symptoms. Depression also influences the availability of social support due to the social isolation and withdrawal induced by the disorder. Furthermore, depression contributes to cognitive distortions and irrational beliefs found to impact on alcohol use relapse.[195] On the other hand, patients with primary major depression may resort to heavy alcohol use in an attempt to alleviate depressive symptoms.

- Mediates the effect of stress on alcohol relapse

- Impacts on adaptational capacity which predicts relapse

- Impairs coping skills

- Impairs self-efficacy

- Influences availability of social support

- Causes cognitive distortion

- Causes irrational beliefs

Table 30
Depression as risk factor for alcohol relapse

- Educate about the course and prognosis of major depression and alcoholism
- Optimize antidepressant treatment using therapeutic doses of the medications
- Treat residual and recurring symptoms of depression
- Educate about long-term effects of the medications
- Educate about the influence of alcohol use on depression and that of depression on alcohol relapse
- Educate about the necessity for medication and the risk of non-compliance
- Help the patient develop a support network
- Help the patient develop effective coping skills
- Correct cognitive distortions and irrational beliefs
- Monitor and address issues related to violent behaviour

Table 31
Maintenance treatment for depressed patients with alcohol dependence

Relapse prevention strategies

Relapse prevention (RP) strategies focus on key issues associated with relapse and long-term recovery. These RP strategies help the patient prepare for the possibility of relapse and hence reduce relapse risk by: (1) identifying and managing individual high-risk relapse factors; (2) identifying and managing early warning signs of relapse; (3) intervening early should a lapse or relapse actually occur; and (4) making broader changes in order to achieve a more balanced lifestyle so that alcohol is not desired.[180]

- **Identifying and managing high-risk situations:** negative emotional states such as anxiety, anger, boredom, emptiness, depression, guilt, shame and loneliness are the most common factors contributing to relapse. Interpersonal situations such as direct or indirect social pressures to drink alcohol or conflicts with another person are the second and third most common precipitants of relapse. The caregiver can help the patient reduce relapse risk by first examining which emotions or interpersonal situations are perceived to be high risk for relapse. Then, specific strategies can be taught related to these high-risk situations. Strategies should be adapted based on the unique features of the high-risk situation for the patient. For example, anger problems with one alcohol-dependent patient may require helping this individual learn to accept and express anger appropriately. Anger problems with another patient may require helping this individual to control anger and rage, and not express it in interpersonal encounters. Boredom for one individual may be a function of lacking interesting hobbies or activities whereas with another, boredom may represent a serious problem in a job in which this person feels underused, underemployed and not challenged.

- **Identifying and managing relapse warning signs:** obvious and subtle warning signs often show prior to an alcohol relapse. These signs show in changes in attitudes, thoughts, feelings and behaviours. For example, a patient's lower motivation may show in an increase in negative attitudes towards recovery or AA which may eventually lead to relapse; or a patient may reduce or stop attending alcoholism treatment and/or AA meetings without first discussing this with someone knowledgeable about his or her situation such as a therapist or AA sponsor. Another common warning sign is putting oneself in high-risk situations such as socializing with old drinking partners. A patient may not be consciously aware of 'a relapse set-up' in this example. Patients can be taught common relapse warning signs and ways to manage these. Patients who have had previous relapse experiences can complete a microanalysis of these experiences in order to become aware of the warning signs that were ignored. Hence, they can learn from past mistakes. Family members can play a helpful role by pointing out warning signs they have observed in the past preceding relapses and by agreeing to let the patient know if they see any current potential relapse warning signs. The following shows a visual representation of the 'road to relapse.'

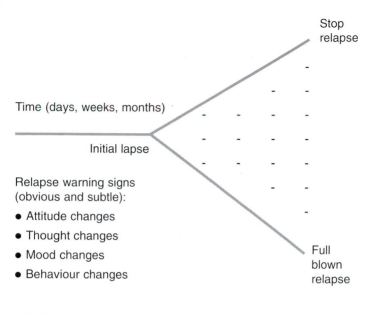

Figure 1
The road to relapse.

- **Managing lapses and relapses:** patients need to
  prepare to intervene early in the process in order to
  prevent a lapse from becoming a relapse, or
  stopping a relapse before it gets out of hand. At the
  fork in the road in Figure 1, the patient's initial
  emotional and cognitive response to a lapse largely
  determines whether there is a return to
  recovery or movement further down the road to a
  full-blown relapse. Patients may feel angry,
  depressed, guilty or shameful following a lapse or
  relapse. They may think 'I'm a failure, I'm incapable
  of changing, I just can't do it, so why even bother

trying', this can fuel the relapse further. Teaching patients to challenge such negative thoughts and rehearsing a plan to interrupt a lapse or relapse ahead of time can prepare patients to take action rather than passively accept that there is nothing they can do.

- **Lifestyle balance:** in addition to specific RP strategies for managing high-risk situations, patients can benefit from broader strategies that reduce stress, improve coping ability or improve health. These include exercise, meditation, focusing on spirituality or focusing on achieving a better balance between 'obligations' in life (shoulds) and 'desires' (wants).

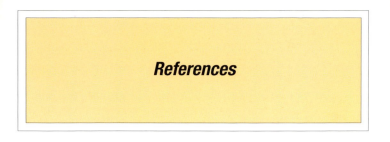

References

1. Regier DA, Farmer ME, Rae DS et al. Comorbidity of mental disorders with alcohol and other drug abuse. Results from the Epidemiologic Catchment Area (ECA) Study [see comments]. *JAMA* 1990; **264**:2511–8.
   Comment in: *JAMA* 1990; **264**: 2549–50, *JAMA* 1991; **265**: 1256–7.

2. Kessler RC, McGonagle KA, Zhao S et al. Lifetime and 12-month prevalence of DSM-III-R psychiatric disorders in the United States. Results from the National Comorbidity Survey. *Archives of General Psychiatry* 1994; **51**: 8–19.

3. Daley DC, Thase ME. *Dual Disorders Recovery Counseling*. Independence Press: Missouri, 1994.

4. Salloum IM, Mezzich JE, Cornelius J et al. Clinical profile of comorbid major depression and alcohol use disorders in an initial psychiatric evaluation. *Comprehensive Psychiatry* 1995; **36**: 260–6.

5. Berkson J. Limitations of the application of fourfold table analysis to hospital data. *Biometric Bulletin* 1946; **2**: 47–53.

6. Steadman HJ, Mulvey EP, Monahan J et al. Violence by people discharged from acute psychiatric inpatient facilities and by others in the same neighborhoods [see comments]. *Archives of General Psychiatry* 1998; **55**: 393–401.
Comment in: *Archives of General Psychiatry* 1998; **55**: 403–4, *Archives of General Psychiatry* 1999; **56**: 193–4.

7. Wettstein RM. *Treatment of Offenders with Mental Disorders.* Guilford Press: New York, 1998.

8. Karper LP, Krystal JH. Pharmacotherapy of violent behavior. Stoff DM, Breiling J, Maser JD (eds). *Handbook of Antisocial Behavior.* John Wiley: New York, 1997: 436–44.

9. Salloum IM, Daley DC, Cornelius JR et al. Disproportionate lethality in psychiatric patients with concurrent alcohol and cocaine abuse [see comments]. *American Journal of Psychiatry* 1996; **153**: 953–5.
Comment in: *American Journal of Psychiatry* 1997; **154**: 888–9.

10. Daley DC. Substance abuse and offending. *Current Opinion in Psychiatry* 1992; **5**: 792–8.

11. Kessler RC, Crum RM, Warner LA et al. Lifetime co-occurrence of DSM-III-R alcohol abuse and dependence with other psychiatric disorders in the National Comorbidity Survey. *Archives of General Psychiatry* 1997; **54**: 313–21.

12. Hanna EZ, Grant BF. Gender differences in DSM-IV alcohol use disorders and major depression as

distributed in the general population: clinical implications. *Comprehensive Psychiatry* 1997; **38**: 202–12.

13. Weissman MM, Myers JK. Clinical depression in alcoholism. *American Journal of Psychiatry* 1980; **137**: 372–3.

14. Helzer JE, Pryzbeck TR. The co-occurrence of alcoholism with other psychiatric disorders in the general population and its impact on treatment. *Journal of Studies on Alcohol* 1988; **49**: 219–24.

15. Willenbring ML. Measurement of depression in alcoholics. *Journal of Studies on Alcohol* 1986; **47**: 367–72.

16. Powell BJ, Penick EC, Othmer E et al. Prevalence of additional psychiatric syndromes among male alcoholics. *Journal of Clinical Psychiatry* 1982; **43**: 404–7.

17. Cadoret R, Winokur G. Depression in alcoholism. *Annals of the New York Academy of Sciences* 1974; **233**: 34–9.

18. Weissman MM, Pottenger M, Kleber H et al. Symptom patterns in primary and secondary depression. A comparison of primary depressives with depressed opiate addicts, alcoholics, and schizophrenics. *Archives of General Psychiatry* 1977; **34**: 854–62.

19. Hesselbrock MN, Meyer RE, Keener JJ. Psychopathology in hospitalized alcoholics. *Archives of General Psychiatry* 1985; **42**: 1050–5.

20. Ross HE, Glaser FB, Germanson T. The prevalence of psychiatric disorders in patients with alcohol and other drug problems. *Archives of General Psychiatry* 1988; **45**: 1023–31.

21. Daley DC, Moss HB, Campbell F. *Dual Disorders: Counseling Clients with Chemical Dependency and Mental Illness.* Hazelden: Minnesota, 1993.

22. Daley DC, Salloum IM, Thase ME. Improving treatment adherence among patients with comorbid psychiatric and substance use disorders. In: O'Connell DF (ed). *Managing the Dually Diagnosed Patient: Current Issues and Clinical Approaches.* Haeworth: New York, in press.

23. Gondolf E. *Psychiatric Response to Family Violence.* Lexington Books: Massachusetts, 1990.

24. Liskow B, Mayfield D, Thiele J. Alcohol and affective disorder: assessment and treatment. *Journal of Clinical Psychiatry* 1982; **43**: 144–7.

25. Schuckit MA. Alcohol and depression: a clinical perspective. *Acta Psychiatrica Scandinavica* 1994; **377**: S28–S32.

26. Cornelius JR, Salloum IM, Mezzich JE et al. Disproportionate suicidality in patients with comorbid major depression and alcoholism. *American Journal of Psychiatry* 1995; **152**: 358–64.

27. Crowe DB, Rosse RB, Sheridan MJ, Deutsch SI. Substance use diagnoses and discharge patterns among psychiatric inpatients. *Hospital and Community Psychiatry* 1991; **42**: 403–5.

28. Preskorn SH, Goodwin DW. Medical management of the depressed alcoholic patient. *International Journal of Psychiatry in Medicine* 1987; **17**: 117–31.

29. Murphy GE, Wetzel RD, Robins E, McEvoy L. Multiple risk factors predict suicide in alcoholism. *Archives of General Psychiatry* 1992; **49**: 459–63.

30. Daley DC, Salloum IM. The family factor. *Professional Counselor* 1996; **11**: 51–6.

31. Moss HB, Salloum IM, Fisher B. Psychoactive substance abuse. In: Hersen M, Ammerman RT et al. (eds) *Handbook of Aggressive and Destructive Behavior in Psychiatric Patients*. Plenum Press: New York, 1994: 175–201.

32. Swanson JW, Holzer CE, Ganju VK, Jono RT. Violence and psychiatric disorder in the community: evidence from the Epidemiologic Catchment Area surveys [published erratum appears in *Hospital and Community Psychiatry* 1991; **42**: 954–5]. *Hospital and Community Psychiatry* 1990; **41**: 761–70.

33. Hoaken PN, Giancola PR, Pihl RO. Executive functions as mediators of alcohol-related aggression. *Alcohol and Alcoholism* 1998; **33**: 47–54.

34. Giancola PR, Mezzich AC, Tarter RE. Disruptive, delinquent and aggressive behavior in female adolescents with a psychoactive substance use disorder: relation to executive cognitive functioning. *Journal of Studies on Alcohol* 1998; **59**: 560–7.

35. Virkkunen M, Goldman D, Linnoila M. Serotonin in alcoholic violent offenders. *Ciba Foundation Symposium* 1996; **194**: 168–77; discussion 177–82.

36. Dabbs JM Jr, Jurkovic GJ, Frady RL. Salivary testosterone and cortisol among late adolescent male offenders. *Journal of Abnormal Child Psychology* 1991; **19**: 469–78.

37. Miczek KA, DeBold JF, van Erp AM, Tornatzky W. Alcohol, GABAA–benzodiazepine receptor complex, and aggression. *Recent Developments in Alcoholism* 1997; **13**: 139–71.

38. Borges G, Cherpitel CJ, Rosovsky H. Male drinking and violence-related injury in the emergency room [see comments]. *Addiction* 1998; **93**: 103–12. Comment in: *Addiction* 1998; **93**: 1261–2.

39. Giancola PR, Zeichner A. The biphasic effects of alcohol on human physical aggression. *Journal of Abnormal Psychology* 1997; **106**: 598–607.

40. White HR. Longitudinal perspective on alcohol use and aggression during adolescence. *Recent Developments in Alcoholism* 1997; **13**: 81–103.

41. Higley JD, Suomi SJ, Linnoila M. A nonhuman primate model of type II alcoholism? Part 2. Diminished social competence and excessive aggression correlates with low cerebrospinal fluid 5-hydroxyindoleacetic acid concentrations. *Alcoholism: Clinical and Experimental Research* 1996; **20**: 643–50.

42. Virkkunen M, Kallio E, Rawlings R et al. Personality profiles and state aggressiveness in Finnish alcoholic, violent offenders, fire setters, and healthy volunteers. *Archives of General Psychiatry* 1994; **51**: 28–33.

43. Cloninger CR, Reich T. Genetic heterogeneity in alcoholism and sociopathy. *Research Publications – Association for Research in Nervous and Mental Disease* 1983; **60**: 145–66.

44. Mann K, Ackermann K, Jung M et al. Aggressiveness, onset of dependence, and treatment outcome in socially well-adapted alcoholics. *Alcohol and Alcoholism* 1998; **33**: 16–19.

45. Schatzberg AF, DeBattista C. Phenomenology and treatment of agitation. *Journal of Clinical Psychiatry* 1999; **60**: S17–S20.

46. Fava M, Rosenbaum JF. Anger attacks in patients with depression. *Journal of Clinical Psychiatry* 1999; **60**: S21–S24.

47. Fava M. Depression with anger attacks. *Journal of Clinical Psychiatry* 1998; **59**: S18–S22.

48. Fava M, Rosenbaum JF, McCarthy M et al. Anger attacks in depressed outpatients and their response to fluoxetine. *Psychopharmacology Bulletin* 1991; **27**: 275–9.

49. Roy A. Suicide and psychiatric patients. *Psychiatric Clinics of North America* 1985; **8**: 227–41.

50. Murphy GE, Wetzel RD. The lifetime risk of suicide in alcoholism. *Archives of General Psychiatry* 1990; **47**: 383–92.

51. Cornelius JR, Salloum IM, Day NL et al. Patterns of suicidality and alcohol use in alcoholics with major depression. *Alcoholism, Clinical and Experimental Research* 1996; **20**: 1451–5.

52. Roy A, Lamparski D, DeJong J et al. Characteristics of alcoholics who attempt suicide. *American Journal of Psychiatry* 1990; **147**: 761–5.

53. Klatsky AL, Armstrong MA. Alcohol use, other traits, and risk of unnatural death: a prospective study. *Alcoholism: Clinical and Experimental Research* 1993; **17**: 1156–62.

54. Coccaro EF, Murphy DL (eds). *Serotonin in Major Psychiatric Disorders.* American Psychiatric Press: Washington DC, 1990.

55. Rosenbaum JF, Fava M, Pava JA et al. Anger attacks in unipolar depression, Part 2: Neuroendocrine correlates and changes following fluoxetine treatment. *American Journal of Psychiatry* 1993; **150**: 1164–8.

56. Higley JD, Suomi SJ, Linnoila M. A nonhuman primate model of type II excessive alcohol consumption? Part 1. Low cerebrospinal fluid 5-hydroxyindoleacetic acid concentrations and diminished social competence correlate with excessive alcohol consumption. *Alcoholism: Clinical and Experimental Research* 1996; **20**: 629–42.

57. Higley JD, Linnoila M. A nonhuman primate model of excessive alcohol intake. Personality and neurobiological parallels of type I- and type II-like alcoholism. *RecentDevelopments in Alcoholism* 1997; **13**: 191–219.

58. Heinz A, Higley JD, Gorey JG et al. In vivo association between alcohol intoxication, aggression, serotonin transporter availability in nonhuman primates. *American Journal of Psychiatry* 1998; **155**: 1023–8.

59. Kavoussi R, Armstead P, Coccaro E. The neurobiology of impulsive aggression. *Psychiatric Clinics of North America*;1997 **20**: 395–403.

60. American Psychiatric Association. *DSM-IV: Diagnostic and Statistical Manual of Mental Disorders*. 4th edn. American Psychiatric Association: Washington DC, 1994.

61. World Health Organization. *The Tenth Revison of the International Classification of Diseases and Related Health Problems* (ICD-10). WHO: Geneva, 1992.

62. American Psychiatric Association. *Substance-related Disorders DSM-IV: Diagnostic and Statistical Manual of Mental Disorders*. 4th edn. American Psychiatric Association: Washington DC, 1994: 175–272.

63. Edwards G, Gross MM. Alcohol dependence: provisional description of a clinical syndrome. *British Medical Journal* 1976; **1**: 1058–61.

64. Nace EP, *The Treatment of Alcoholism*. Brunner/Mazel: New York, 1987.

65. Pattison EM. Clinical approaches to the alcoholic patient. *Psychosomatics* 1986; **27**: 762–7.

66. Galanter M. Network Therapy. In: Galanter M, Kleber HD (eds). *Textbook of Substance Abuse Treatment*. 2nd edn. American Psychiatric Press: Washington DC, 1999: 323–34.

67. Romach MK, Sellers EM. Management of the alcohol withdrawal syndrome. *Annual Review of Medicine* 1991; **42**: 323–40.

68. NIAAA Treatment Handbook Series 4. *Assessing Alcohol Problems: A Guide for Clinicians and Researchers.* NIH Publication No. 95–3745: Rockville, MD, 1995: 573.

69. Sobell MB, Sobell LC. Problem drinkers: Guided Self-Change Treatment. Guilford Press: New York, 1993.

70. Skinner HA, Sheu WJ. Reliability of alcohol use indices: The Lifetime Drinking History and the MAST. *Journal of Studies on Alcohol* 1982; **43**: 1157–70.

71. Horn JL, Wanberg KW, Foster FM. The Alcohol Use Inventory. Psych Systems: Baltimore, MD, 1983.

72. Annis HM. Inventory of Drinking Situations. Addictions Research Foundation of Ontario: Toronto, 1982.

73. McLellan AT, Alterman AI, Cacciloa J et al. A new measure of substance abuse treatment: Initial studies of the Treatment Service Review. *Journal of Nervous and Mental Disease* 1992; **180**: 101–10.

74. Miller WR, Marlatt GA. Comprehensive Drinker Profile Manual Supplement for Use with Brief Drinker Profile, Follow-up Drinker Profile, Collateral Interview Form. Psychological Assesement Resources: Odessa, FL, 1987.

75. Mayfield D, McLeod G, Hall P. The CAGE questionnaire: validation of a new alcoholism screening instrument. *American Journal of Psychiatry:* 1974; **131**: 1121–3.

76. Selzer ML. The Michigan Alcoholism Screening Test: the quest for a new diagnostic instrument. *American Journal of Psychiatry* 1971; **127**: 1653–8.

77. Saunders JB, Aasland OG, Babor TF et al. Development of the Alcohol Use Disorders Identification Test (AUDIT): WHO collaborative project on early detection of persons with harmful alcohol consumption: II. *Addiction* 1993; **88**: 791–804.

78. Skinner HA, Allen BA. Alcohol dependence syndrome: measurement and validation. *Journal of Abnormal Psychology* 1982; **91**: 199–209.

79. Stockwell T, Murphy D, Hodgson R. The severity of alcohol dependence questionnaire: its use, reliability and validity. *British Journal of Addiction* 1983; **78**: 145–55.

80. First MB, Spitzer RL, Gibbon M, Williams JB. *Structured Clinical Interview for DSM-IV–Axis I Disorders.* New York State Psychiatric Institute: New York, 1994.

81. Hasin DS, Trautman KD, Miele GM et al. Psychiatric Research Interview for Substance and Mental Disorders (PRISM): reliability for substance abusers. *American Journal of Psychiatry* 1996; **153**: 1195–201.

82. Spitzer RL, Williams JW et al. Utility of a new procedure for diagnosing mental disorders in primary care: the PRIME-MD 1000 study. *Journal of the American Medical Association* 1994; **272**: 1749–56.

83. Sobell LC, Sobell MB, Leo GI, Cancilla A. Reliability of a timeline method: assessing normal drinkers' reports of recent drinking and a comparative

evaluation across several populations. *British Journal of Addiction* 1988; **83**: 393–402.

84. McLellan AT, Luborsky L, Woody GE, O'Brien CP. An improved diagnostic evaluation instrument for substance abuse patients. The addiction severity index. *Journal of Nervous and Mental Disease* 1980; **168**: 26–33.

85. Monti PM, Rohsenow DJ, Abrams DB et al. Development of a behavior analytically derived alcohol-specific role-play assessment instrument. *Journal of Studies on Alcohol* 1993; **54**: 710–21.

86. Miller WR, Tonigan JS, Longabaugh R. *The Drinker Inventory of Consequences (DrInC): An Instrument for Assessing Adverse Consequences of Alcohol Abuse. Test Manual.* US Government Printing Office, NIAAA Project MATCH Monograph Series. Vol. 4. NIH Pub. No.95–3911: Washington DC, 1995.

87. Sullivan JT, Sykora K, Schneiderman J et al. Assessment of alcohol withdrawal: the revised clinical institute withdrawal assessment for alcohol scale (CIWA-Ar). *British Journal of Addiction* 1989; **84**: 1353–7.

88. Salloum IM, Cornelius JR, Daley DC, Thase ME. The utility of diazepam loading in the treatment of alcohol withdrawal among psychiatric inpatients. *Psychopharmacology Bulletin* 1995; **31**: 305–10.

89. Nolen-Hoeksema S, Morrow J, Fredrickson BL. Response styles and the duration of episodes of depressed mood. *Journal of Abnormal Psychology* 1993; **102**: 20–8.

90. Cooper ML, Russell M, George WH. Coping, expectancies, and alcohol abuse: a test of social learning formulations. *Journal of Abnormal Psychology* 1988; **97**: 218–30.

91. Farber PD, Khavari KA, Douglas FM. A factor analytic study of reasons for drinking: empirical validation of positive and negative reinforcement dimensions. *Journal of Consulting and Clinical Psychology* 1980; **48**: 780–1.

92. Gjerde PF, Westenberg P. Dysphoric adolescents as young adults: A prospective study of the psychological sequelae of depressed mood in adolescence. *Journal of Research on Adolescence* 1998; **8**: 377–402.

93. Zlotnick C, Shea MT, Pilkonis PA et al. Gender, type of treatment, dysfunctional attitudes, social support, life events and depressive symptoms over naturalistic follow-up. *American Journal of Psychiatry* 1996; **153**: 1021–7.

94. Simpson HB, Nee JC, Endicott J. First-episode major depression. Few sex differences in course. *Archives of General Psychiatry* 1997; **54**: 633–9.

95. Williams JB, Spitzer RL, Linzer M et al. Gender differences in depression in primary care. *American Journal of Obstetrics and Gynecology* 1995; **173**: 654–9.

96. Schuckit MA. The relationship between alcohol problems, substance abuse, and psychiatric syndromes. In: Widiger AT, Frances JA, Pincus HA et al. *DSM-IV Sourcebook. Vol. 1*. American Psychiatric Association: Washington DC; 1994: 45–66.

97. Hamilton M. Rating depressive patients. *Journal of Clinical Psychiatry* 1960; **41**: 21–4.

98. Beck AT, Beamesderfer A. Assessment of depression: the depression inventory. *Modern Problems of Pharmacopsychiatry* 1974; **7**: 151–69.

99. Brown SA, Inaba RK, Gillin JC et al. Alcoholism and affective disorder: clinical course of depressive symptoms. *American Journal of Psychiatry* 1995; **152**: 45–52.

100. Cornelius JR, Salloum IM, Ehler JG et al. Fluoxetine in depressed alcoholics. A double-blind, placebo-controlled trial [see comments]. *Archives of General Psychiatry* 1997; **54**: 700–5. Comment in: *Archives of General Psychiatry* 1997; **54**: 691–4.

101. Mason BJ, Kocsis JH, Ritvo EC et al. A double-blind, placebo-controlled trial of desipramine for primary alcohol dependence stratified on the presence or absence of major depression. *Journal of the American Medical Association* 1996; **275**: 761–7.

102. Murphy GE, Wetzel RD, Robins E, McEvoy L. Multiple risk factors predict suicide in alcoholism. *Archives of General Psychiatry* 1992; **49**: 459–63.

103. Lion JR. Aggression. In: Kaplan HI, Sadock BJ (eds). *Comprehensive Textbook of Psychiatry*. 6th edn. Williams & Wilkins: Baltimore, 1995: 310–17.

104. National Institute on Alcohol Abuse and Alcoholism (NIAAA). *Motivational Enhancement Therapy Manual: A Clinical Research Guide for Therapists Treating Individuals with Alcohol Abuse and Dependence*.

Project MATCH Monograph Series Volume 2. US Department of Health and Human Services: Rockville, MD, 1995.

105. Bien TH, Miller WR, Toniga JS. Brief interventions for alcohol problems: a review. *Addiction* 1993; **88**: 315–36.

106. Miller WR, Benefield TG, Tonigan JS. Enhancing motivation for change in problem drinking: a controlled comparison of two therapist styles. *Journal of Consulting and Clinical Psychology* 1993; **61**: 455–61.

107. Saunders B, Wilkinson C, Phillips M. The impact of a brief motivational intervention with opiate users attending a methadone program. *Addiction* 1995; **90**: 415–24.

108. Smith DE, Heckemeyer CM, Kratt PP, Mason DA. Motivational interviewing to improve adherence to a behavioral weight-control program for older obese women with NIDDM. *Diabetes Care* 1997; **20**: 52–4.

109. Daley DC, Zuckoff A. Improving compliance with the initial outpatient session among discharged inpatient dual diagnosis clients. *Social Work* 1998; **43**: 470–3.

110. Daley DC, Zuckoff A. *Improving Treatment Compliance: Counseling and System Strategies for Substance Use and Dual Disorders*. Hazelden: Minnesota, 1999.

111. Daley DC, Salloum IM, Zuckoff A et al. Increasing treatment adherence among outpatients with depression and cocaine dependence: results of a pilot study. *American Journal of Psychiatry* 1998; **155**: 1611–13.

112. Rosenthal RN, Perkel C, Singh P et al. A pilot open randomized trial of valproate and phenobarbital in the treatment of acute alcohol withdrawal. *American Journal on Addictions* 1998; **7**: 189–97.

113. Miller WR, Rollnick S. *Motivational Interviewing: Preparing People to Change Addictive Behavior*. Guilford Press: New York, 1991.

114. Hester RK, Miller WR. *Handbook of Alcoholism Treatment Approaches*: Effective Alternatives. 2nd edn. Allyn and Bacon: Massachusetts, 1995.

115. McGrath PJ, Nunes EV, Stewart JW et al. Imipramine treatment of alcoholics with primary depression: a placebo-controlled clinical trial. *Archives of General Psychiatry* 1996; **53**: 232–40.

116. Weiss RD, Najavits LM. Overview of treatment modalities for dual diagnosis patients: pharmacotherapy, psychotherapy, and 12-step programs. In: Kranzler HH, Rounsaville BJ (eds). *Dual Diagnosis and Treatment: Substance Abuse and Comorbid Medical and Psychiatric Disorders*. 13th edn. Marcel Dekker: New York, 1998: 107–37.

117. Ciraulo DA, Shader RI. *Clinical Manual of Chemical Dependence*. American Psychiatric Press: Washington DC,1991.

118. Fuller RK, Gordis E. Refining the treatment of alcohol withdrawal [editorial; comment]. *Journal of the American Medical Association* 1994; **272**: 557–8. Comment in: *Journal of the American Medical Association* 1994; **272**: 519–23.

119. Sellers EM, Naranjo CA, Harrison M et al. Diazepam loading: simplified treatment of alcohol withdrawal.

Clinical Pharmacology and Therapeutics 1983; **34**: 822–6.

120. American Psychiatric Association. Mood Disorders. In: *DSM-IV: Diagnostic and Statistical Manual of Mental Disorders*. 4th edn. American Psychiatric Association: Washington DC, 1994: 317–91.

121. Salloum IM, Cornelius JR, Thase ME et al. Naltrexone utility in depressed alcoholics. *Psychopharmacology Bulletin* 1998; **34**: 111–15.

122. Litten RZ, Allen JP. Pharmacologic treatment of alcoholics with collateral depression: issues and future directions. *Psychopharmacology Bulletin* 1998; **34**: 107–10.

123. Rounsaville BJ, Dolinsky ZS, Babor TF, Meyer RE. Psychopathology as a predictor of treatment outcome in alcoholics. *Archives of General Psychiatry* 1987; **44**: 505–13.

124. Anton RF. Neurobehavioural basis for the pharmacotherapy of alcoholism: current and future directions. *Alcohol and Alcoholism* 1996; **31**: S43–S53.

125. Lewis MJ. Alcohol reinforcement and neuropharmacological therapeutics. *Alcohol and Alcoholism* 1996; **31**: S17–S25.

126. Meyer RE. Prospects for a rational pharmacotherapy of alcoholism. *Journal of Clinical Psychiatry* 1989; **50**: 403–12.

127. Lejoyeux M. Use of serotonin (5-hydroxytryptamine) reuptake inhibitors in the treatment of alcoholism. *Alcohol and Alcoholism* 1996; **1**: S69–S75.

128. Ciraulo DA, Barnhill JG, Jaffe JH. Clinical pharmaco-kinetics of imipramine and desipramine in alcoholics and normal volunteers. *Clinical Pharmacology and Therapeutics* 1988; **43**: 509–18.

129. Naranjo CA, Sellers EM, Sullivan JT et al. The serotonin uptake inhibitor citalopram attenuates ethanol intake. *Clinical Pharmacology and Therapeutics* 1987; **41**: 266–74.

130. Naranjo CA, Bremner KE, Lanctot KL. Effects of citalopram and a brief psychosocial intervention on alcohol intake, dependence and problems. *Addiction* 1995; **90**: 87–99.

131. Angst J, Angst F, Stassen HH. Suicide risk in patients with major depressive disorder. *Journal of Clinical Psychiatry* 1999; **60**: S57–S62; discussion S75–S76, S113–S116.

132. Thase ME. Depression, sleep, and antidepressants. *Journal of Clinical Psychiatry* 1998; **59**: S55–S65.

133. Gillin JC, Smith TL, Irwin M et al. Increased pressure for rapid eye movement sleep at time of hospital admission predicts relapse in nondepressed patients with primary alcoholism at 3-month follow-up. *Archives of General Psychiatry* 1994; **51**: 189–97.

134. Salloum IM, Cornelius JR, Daley DC et al. Naltrexone fluoxetine medication interaction in depressed alcoholics: Preliminary results. *Alcoholism: Clinical and Experimental Research* 1999; **23**: 47A.

135. Litten RZ, Allen J, Fertig J. Pharmacotherapies for alcohol problems: a review of research with focus on developments since 1991 [see comments].

Alcoholism: Clinical and Experimental Research 1996; **20**: 859–76.
Comment in: *Alcoholism: Clinical and Experimental Research* 1997; **21**: 380.

136. Anton RF, Kranzler HR, Meyer RE. Neurobehavioral aspects of the pharmacotherapy of alcohol dependence. *Clinical Neuroscience* 1995; **3**: 145–54.

137. Fuller RK, Branchey L, Brightwell DR et al. Disulfiram treatment of alcoholism. A Veterans Administration cooperative study. *Journal of the American Medical Association* 1986; **256**: 1449–55.

138. Chick J, Gough K, Falkowski W et al. Disulfiram treatment of alcoholism. *British Journal of Psychiatry* 1992; **161**: 84–9.

139. Salloum IM, Cornelius JR. Management of side effects of drugs used in treatment of alcoholism and drug abuse. In: Balon R (ed.). *Practical Management of the Side Effects of Psychotropic Drugs*. Marcel Dekker: New York, 1999: 169–97.

140. Croop RS, Faulkner EB, Labriola DF. The safety profile of naltrexone in the treatment of alcoholism. Results from a multicenter usage study. The Naltrexone Usage Study Group. *Archives of General Psychiatry* 1997; **54**: 1130–5.

141. Virkkunen M, Linnoila M. Serotonin in early-onset alcoholism. *Recent Developments in Alcoholism* 1997; **13**: 173–89.

142. Fava M, Rosenbaum JF. Psychopharmacology of pathologic aggression. *Harvard Review of Psychiatry* 1993; **1**: 244–6.

143. Hollander E. Managing aggressive behavior in patients with obsessive–compulsive disorder and borderline personality disorder. *Journal of Clinical Psychiatry* 1999; **60**: S38–S44.

144. McDougle CJ, Naylor ST, Cohen DJ et al. A double-blind, placebo-controlled study of fluvoxamine in adults with autistic disorder [see comments]. *Archives of General Psychiatry* 1996; **53**: 1001–8. Comment in: *Archives of General Psychiatry* 1996; **53**: 980–3, *Archives of General Psychiatry* 1998; **55**: 643–4.

145. Davanzo PA, Belin TR, Widawski MH, King BH. Paroxetine treatment of aggression and self-injury in persons with mental retardation. *American Journal of Mental Retardation* 1998; **102**: 427–37.

146. Vartiainen H, Tiihonen J, Putkonen A et al. Citalopram, a selective serotonin reuptake inhibitor, in the treatment of aggression in schizophrenia. *Acta Psychiatrica Scandinavica* 1995; **91**: 348–51.

147. Lavine R. Psychopharmacological treatment of aggression and violence in the substance using population. *Journal of Psychoactive Drugs* 1997; **29**: 321–9.

148. Tardiff K. The current state of psychiatry in the treatment of violent patients. *Archives of General Psychiatry* 1992; **49**: 493–9.

149. Spreat S, Behar D, Reneski B, Miazzo P. Lithium carbonate for aggression in mentally retarded persons. *Comprehensive Psychiatry* 1989; **30**: 505–11.

150. Linnoila M, Virkkunen M, Roy A et al. Violence and suicidality: perspectives in clinical and psychobiological research. *Clinical and Experimental Psychiatry. Vol. 3.* Brunner/Mazel: New York, 1990: 218–41.

151. Corrigan PW, Yudofsky SC, Silver JM. Pharmacological and behavioral treatments for aggressive psychiatric inpatients. *Hospital and Community Psychiatry* 1993; **44**: 125–33.

152. Pfeffer CR, Jiang H, Domeshek LJ. Buspirone treatment of psychiatrically hospitalized prepubertal children with symptoms of anxiety and moderately severe aggression. *Journal of Child and Adolescent Psychopharmacology* 1997; **7**: 145–55.

153. Hector RI. The use of clozapine in the treatment of aggressive schizophrenia. *Canadian Journal of Psychiatry – Revue Canadienne de Psychiatrie* 1998; **43**: 466–72.

154. Glazer WM, Dickson RA. Clozapine reduces violence and persistent aggression in schizophrenia. *Journal of Clinical Psychiatry* 1998; **59**: S8–S14.

155. Fava M. Psychopharmacologic treatment of pathologic aggression. *Psychiatric Clinics of North America* 1997; **20**: 427–51.

156. Potenza MN, Holmes JP, Kanes SJ, McDougle CJ. Olanzapine treatment of children, adolescents, and adults with pervasive developmental disorders: an open-label pilot study. *Journal of Clinical Psychopharmacology* 1999; **19**: 37–44.

157. John V, Rapp M, Pies R. Aggression, agitation, and mania with olanzapine [letter]. *Canadian Journal of Psychiatry - Revue Canadienne de Psychiatrie* 1998; **43**: 1054.

158. National Institute on Alcohol Abuse and Alcoholism (NIAAA). *Cognitive-Behavioral Coping Skills Therapy Manual: A Clinical Research Guide for Therapists Treating Individuals with Alcohol Abuse and Dependence.* Project MATCH Monograph Series Volume 3. US Department of Health and Human Services: Rockville, MD, 1995.

159. National Institute on Alcohol Abuse and Alcoholism (NIAAA). *Twelve Step Facilitation Therapy Manual: A Clinical Research Guide for Therapists Treating Individuals with Alcohol Abuse and Dependence.* Project MATCH Monograph Series Volume 1. US Department of Health and Human Services: Rockville, MD, 1995.

160. Edwards MR, Steinglass P. Family therapy treatment outcomes for alcoholism. *Journal of Marital and Family Therapy* 1995; **21**: 475–509.

161. Stanton MD, Shadish WR. Outcome, attrition, and family-couples treatment for drug abuse: a meta-analysis and review of the controlled, comparative studies. *Psychological Bulletin* 1997; **122**: 170–91.

162. Meyers RJ, Smith JE. *Clinical Guide to Alcohol Treatment: The Community Reinforcement Approach.* Guilford Press: New York, 1995.

163. Szapocznik J, Perez-Vidal A, Brickman AL et al. Engaging adolescent drug abusers and their families

in treatment: a strategic structural systems approach. *Journal of Consulting and Clinical Psychology* 1988; **56**: 552–7.

164. O'Farrell TG. *Treating Alcohol Problems: Marital and Family Interventions*. Guilford Press: New York, 1993.

165. Garrett J, Landau-Stanton J, Stanton MD et al. ARISE: a method for engaging reluctant alcohol-and drug-dependent individuals in treatment. *Journal of Substance Abuse Treatment* 1997; **14**: 235–48.

166. Klerman GL, Weissman MM, Rounsaville BJ, Chevron ES. *Interpersonal Psychotherapy of Depression*. Basic Books: New York, 1984.

167. Beck AR, Rush AJ, Shaw BF. *Cognitive Therapy of Depression*. Guilford Press: New York, 1979.

168. Beck A, Freeman A & Associates. *Cognitive Therapy of Personality Disorders*. Guilford Press: New York, 1990.

169. Linehan MM. *Skills Training Manual for Treating Borderline Personality Disorder*. Guilford Press: New York, 1993.

170. Linehan MM. *Cognitive-Behavioral Treatment of Borderline Personality Disorder*. Guilford Press: New York, 1993.

171. Marques JK, Day DM, Nelson C, Miner MH. The Sex Offender Treatment and Evaluation Project: California's Relapse Prevention Program. In: Laws DR (ed). *Relapse Prevention with Sex Offenders*. Guilford Press: New York, 1989: 247–67.

172. Marshall WL, Hudson SM, Ward T. Sexual deviance. In: Wilson PH (ed). *Principles and Practice of Relapse Prevention.* Guilford Press: New York, 1992: 235–54.

173. Substance Abuse and Mental Health Services Administration. *Counselor's Manual for Relapse Prevention with Chemically Dependent Criminal Offenders.* Criminal Justice Subseries, Volume II edition. US Department of Health and Human Services: New York, 1996.

174. Bradley BD. *The Domestic Violence Sourcebook: Everything You Need to Know.* Lowell House: California, 1996.

175. Dutton DG. *The Abusive Personality: Violence and Control in Intimate Relationships.* Guilford Press: New York, 1998.

176. Hampton RL (ed). *Family Violence.* 2nd edn. Sage Publications: California, 1999.

177. Carnes PJ. *The Sexual Addiction.* CompCare Publications: Minnesota, 1983.

178. Thase ME. Long-term nature of depression. *Journal of Clinical Psychiatry* 1999; **60**: S3–S9; discussion S31–S35.

179. Vaillant GE. *The Natural History of Alcoholism Revisited.* Harvard University Press: Massachusetts, 1995.

180. Daley DC, Marlatt GA. Relapse prevention. In: Lowinson JH, Ruiz P, Millman RB, Langrod JG (eds). *Substance Abuse: A Comprehensive Textbook.* 3rd edn. Williams & Wilkins: Baltimore, MD, 1997: 458–66.

181. Akiskal H. Mood disorders. In: Kaplan HI, Sadock BJ (eds). *Comprehensive Textbook of Psychiatry*. 6th edn. Vol. 2. Williams & Wilkins: Baltimore, MD,1995: 1123–52.

182. Angst J. Fortnightly review. A regular review of the long-term follow up of depression. *British Medical Journal* 1997; **315**: 1143–6.

183. Kupfer DJ, Frank E, Perel JM et al. Five-year outcome for maintenance therapies in recurrent depression. *Archives of General Psychiatry* 1992; **49**: 769–73.

184. Frank E, Kupfer DJ, Perel JM et al. Three-year outcomes for maintenance therapies in recurrent depression. *Archives of General Psychiatry* 1990; **47**: 1093–9.

185. Kupfer DJ. Management of recurrent depression. *Journal of Clinical Psychiatry* 1993; **54** S29–S33; discussion S34–S35.

186. Post RM. Mood disorders: somatic treatment. In: Kaplan HI, Sadock BJ (eds). *Comprehensive Textbook of Psychiatry*. 6th edn. Vol. 2. Williams & Wilkins: Baltimore, MD, 1995: 1152–78.

187. Gonzales LR, Lewinsohn PM, Clarke GN. Longitudinal follow-up of unipolar depressives: an investigation of predictors of relapse. *Journal of Consulting and Clinical Psychology* 1985; **53**: 461–9.

188. Maj M, Veltro F, Pirozzi R et al. Pattern of recurrence of illness after recovery from an episode of major depression: a prospective study. *American Journal of Psychiatry* 1992; **149**: 795–800.

189. Post RM. Transduction of psychosocial stress into the neurobiology of recurrent affective disorder. *American Journal of Psychiatry* 1992; **149**: 999–1010.

190. Mueller TI, Leon AC, Keller MB et al. Recurrence after recovery from major depressive disorder during 15 years of observational follow-up. *American Journal of Psychiatry* 1999; **156**: 1000–6.

191. Lin EH, Katon WJ, von Korff M et al. Relapse of depression in primary care. Rate and clinical predictors [see comments]. *Archives of Family Medicine* 1998; **7**: 443–9.
Comment in: *Archives of Family Medicine* 1998; **7**: 462–4.

192. Vaillant GE. A long-term follow-up of male alcohol abuse. *Archives of General Psychiatry* 1996 **53**: 243–9.

193. Brown SA, Vik PW, McQuaid JR et al. Severity of psychosocial stress and outcome of alcoholism treatment. *Journal of Abnormal Psychology* 1990; **99**: 344–8.

194. Brown SA, Vik PW, Patterson TL et al. Stress, vulnerability and adult alcohol relapse. *Journal of Studies on Alcohol* 1995; **56**: 538–45.

195. Camatta CD, Nagoshi CT. Stress, depression, irrational beliefs, and alcohol use and problems in a college student sample. *Alcoholism: Clinical and Experimental Research* 1995; **19**: 142–6.

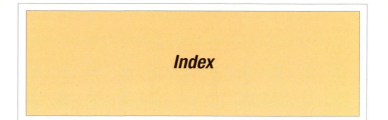
Index